M.E., Chronic Fatigue Syndrome and Fibromyalgia

The Reverse Therapy™ Approach

Dr John Eaton Ph.D.

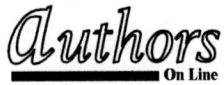

Visit us online at www.authorsonline.co.uk

Contents

Introduction

Carrie came to see me after suffering from Chronic Fatigue Syndrome (CFS) for eighteen years.[1] When she entered my office she was thirty-eight years old but looked fifty-five. She was terribly depressed. But what was worse than the depression were her symptoms. She was in constant pain from the muscle aches that gave her no rest. She was plagued by headaches and nausea and each time she stood up it was all she could do to preserve her balance. This was the reason she walked everywhere with the aid of two walking sticks. But worst of all was the fatigue. She told me that hardly a day went by when she didn't feel drained of energy. She felt so tired that all she wanted to do was sleep and then, when she got up, to go back to bed and try to sleep all over again. But sleep gave her no rest for she often felt as tired afterwards as she did before. She told me that she had no life, for one wearying day was much like the others with nothing to look forward to but pain and exhaustion. She had no job and although she had children and a marriage, she had little involvement with them beyond the small amount of time she could spare for them in between her fatigue spells.

Four sessions of Reverse Therapy later and Carrie had, as she put it, 'got my life back'. Her symptoms were gone. To her family's astonishment she had started running for twenty minutes a day (and had started to lose weight), was going to parties, organising shopping trips and driving everywhere. What was more, she was starting to look for a job and hoped to fulfil her life-long dream of working in some capacity in animal care. She was entirely free of pain and her energy level seemed to her to be sky-high. (It was probably normal but after years of fatigue, to her, it felt that way!)

With great emotion on both sides, I told Carrie that her treatment was over and she could get on with the rest of her life.

How was this cure possible? To give an explanation for this is the reason this book was written. If you are a reader who has been

---

[1] All clients mentioned in this book are based on actual cases. However, all names, and many significant details, have been changed to preserve anonymity.

diagnosed as suffering from Chronic Fatigue Syndrome, M.E. (Myalgic Encephalomyelitis), Fibromyalgia or so-called Post-Viral Fatigue Syndrome, then you too can discover how Reverse Therapy can return you to health.

Reverse Therapy is essentially a simple process in which people learn to listen to their Bodymind and understand the deeper reasons why Bodymind needs to produce symptoms. This process of enlightenment goes side-by-side with dropping the many wrong and confused ideas people have been given about illness, recovery and health.

The misinformation given to sufferers with these illnesses – for example, that they are caused by unknown viral infections, or (the opposite view) that they are disguised forms of Depression – is one reason the cure has been so long in arriving. For neither view is correct. One of my aims in writing this book is to dispel the mystery surrounding these conditions and explain the true cause. Once the cause is understood then the remedy becomes plain.

Many people with M.E./CFS or FMS lead lives of fear, frustration and despair because not only are they struggling to cope with their condition, but also with widespread ignorance and lack of any available help. Too often their illnesses are dismissed or, if they are taken seriously, sufferers are told there is nothing that can be done for them.

The notion that symptoms of M.E./Chronic Fatigue Syndrome and Fibromyalgia are 'all in the mind' is one example of ignorance. As we shall see, this is very far from being the case. The symptoms are in fact created by glandular changes in the body and are very real indeed! These hormonal changes are, in turn, triggered by signals from the Emotional brain, which is the core mechanism of Bodymind.

One important theme of this book – in fact it is a key to understanding Reverse Therapy – is that we must learn to discard the over-emphasis on 'Headmind' in our culture and instead pay more attention to 'Bodymind', the emotive, protective function which works through glandular changes in the body to flag up distress. The real solution to the conditions mentioned above, as well as many others, lies in realising that they are neither mental nor viral in origin but ways in which Bodymind seeks to communicate to us about threatening situations and to encourage us to resolve them. When we do this the essential conditions for returning health are restored.

I have been learning, developing and experimenting with the ideas in this book since 1996. I would like to make it clear that none of the ingredients that go to make up Reverse Therapy are new, although the synthesis is, as well as the unique, step-by-step treatment process.

I have learned much from my many teachers, who have helped me on the way. These include: Ray Keedy, John Grinder, Bill O'Hanlon, Stephen Gilligan, Ernest Rossi and, standing behind us all, Milton Erickson. I have also learnt a great deal from Wilhelm Reich, Fritz Perls and Eugene Gendlin. To all these men I owe a great debt of thanks for, without them, Reverse Therapy could not have been born.

Chapter 1

The Origins of Reverse Therapy

In this chapter you will learn:

> *How Reverse Therapy grew out of my personal experiences*
> *How Milton Erickson and Dr Ernest Rossi influenced me*
> *Where Bodymind communication and the idea of 'listening to symptoms' came from*
> *The difference between Reverse Therapy and psychotherapy*

My own experience of Bodymind

Reverse Therapy is an innovative Bodymind healing process which 'listens' to symptoms in order to establish what needs to happen for a person to be restored to health. The focus of this approach lies in communicating with Bodymind – the unconscious intelligence of the body.

Reverse Therapy is not fixed; it is still evolving. But when I came to give the name 'Reverse Therapy' to this process in 2002 several elements were already in the mixture. These were:

- My own personal experiences
- Ericksonian therapy
- Methods for communicating with Bodymind
- Symptom-focused work
- Psychobiology

All these elements will be described in their proper place

I begin with an experience which first brought home to me the mystery of Bodymind and the way in which it uses symptoms to communicate that something is wrong. This experience was perhaps the most frightening and disturbing of my entire life. It was also profoundly educational.

I was then in the third year of employment as a Printer's Apprentice and I was eighteen years old. I had been more or less thrown out of my grammar school at fifteen for misbehaviour and my father, from the old-fashioned working-class, thought it better anyway that I learned a trade. Glad to be away from the hated school, I readily agreed. The first year or so was fine but then I awoke to the fact that I found the work boring. Setting up and proof-reading type, and then clearing it all away again, soon became monotonous. Moreover, I had little in common with the other printers. I was overly-serious and very studious while most of them had little interest in ideas. I was an idealist where (it seemed to me) they were grindingly materialistic. In short, I was not only regarded (justifiably) as a useless printer but also as a dreamer. I began to see my apprenticeship as a horrible mistake. At that time, an apprentice signed 'Articles' which bound the apprentice to the employer for six years. I could only be released from them with the agreement of the employer. I sought my father's help and he flatly refused to intercede. I wanted to go back to college, which he saw as a waste of time and would mean giving up the promise of a solid trade. Rather like David Copperfield in the blacking factory, I reluctantly settled down to the daily grind.

I became depressed. As I shall explain later, 'de-pression' is designed in some cases to cover over uncomfortable feelings we cannot deal with. In my case this feeling was a great fear that not only was I wasting my life, but to leave my job would leave me without money and possibly without a home. I felt trapped and, slowly, the depressed state got worse. One Monday, at precisely 11.50 a.m., while I was staring at the clock that hung over the Composing Room I experienced a massive panic attack. It seemed to me that something alien was rising up through my body with tremendous force. I couldn't breathe and my heart was beating so fast I really thought I was going to die. What was worse, my body was shaking uncontrollably as sweat poured off me. The whole episode could not have lasted more than two minutes yet it seemed to go on for an eternity. I was still staring at the clock and noticed the hands did not seem to move.

At that time I assumed that people whose bodies did this to them must be mad and I took steps to act as if everything was normal (I was hidden out of sight of most people anyway, behind my composing desk). After a while the panic faded away and I eventually went home. From then on, every day, I dreaded the approach to mid-day. For I knew that, as soon as the clock showed 11.50 a.m., the panic attack would return. First would come the uprising feeling, like a pressure cooker coming to the boil, then the shaking would start. I was helpless to avoid it, or control it, and was terrified. Eventually, after a week of this, the Foreman came over to me and asked if I was 'all right'. Realising my secret was out, I told him my dreadful story (I omitted the detail about the clock). Surprisingly, he was very sympathetic and told me to take a few days off and see a doctor.

I went to see the GP the next day. When he heard of my condition he took the trouble to spend a half-hour with me (he was a very busy man and had held up his surgery just for me). He explained what a panic attack was and told me that it was typically the outcome after a long period of stress. He then told me about his experiences as a member of a bomber aircrew during the war. He and all his friends in the crew were barely out of their teens. Yet almost nightly they went through the terror of being shot at, possibly blown up or set on fire, or bailing out to be drowned in the North Sea. He had seen many of his friends break down from fear or trauma, as he had once himself. He explained that many of them had had no choice but to carry on but that I did have a choice. If I was unhappy then it was important that I made the right decision if I was to get my emotional health back. He told me that he would not prescribe any drugs for me as they would not solve the real problem. He encouraged me to think over what it was I really wanted to do and get on with making it happen, if not now then later.

I am deeply grateful to that very enlightened doctor for he probably saved me from years of illness. This time I spoke earnestly to my parents and, after much persuasion by my mother, my father reluctantly agreed to speak to my employer. The next term I enrolled on a college course and, after a few weeks in a new and more rewarding life as a student, the panic attacks ceased.

I did not realise the significance of this experience until years later, after I got on the path that led to Reverse Therapy. At that time it just seemed to be one of those inexplicable and disturbing things my body did when I was stressed. I did not see then that my Bodymind had been attempting to communicate with me for some time before the panic attacks started by sending me warning 'messages' in the form of the emotions of sadness and frustration. Because I was too ignorant to recognise these feelings for what they were, because no one around me was able to help me deal with them, and because I was afraid of acting on my own, I simply repressed them. But Bodymind is stronger than Headmind and all that denial did was to create an explosion of fear in the form of panic. Only by taking my doctor's advice and acting on the needs that underpinned the original emotions could the panic be dispelled. It was years later before I understood this subtle logic behind the symptoms.

My path towards Reverse Therapy

The path of discovery that led to Reverse Therapy really begins at the end of the 1980s when I first got interested in therapy. At the time, I was myself undergoing therapy for problems that arose with the temporary break-down of my marriage (I had still not learned to recognise and deal with my emotions properly even at that time!). I was impressed by my therapist, a guy called Nigel. He had an air of serenity allied to common-sense and emotional shrewdness that encouraged frankness. He would frequently tell me that my emotions were powerful expressions of my deepest desires, experiences and personal truths and that I alone could do the work of understanding them and resolving them through my actions and words. But what really intrigued me were his questions. He had the knack of asking questions that really forced me to re-think my assumptions about things I had always taken for granted. For example, I remember telling him once that I couldn't help my low moods, they 'just happened' (I often got depressed when I was younger and had been told by my mother it was 'the family curse', carrying the implication that there was little I could about it). Immediately, Nigel asked:

'Yes, and when they are about to happen, how do you know that is the case?'

This question flummoxed me and I didn't know how to answer it. In fact it took a few days for me to make sense of the question and when I did, I realised there was a subtle process of learning that had been going on throughout my life up to that point. Somehow I had learned to have depressed moods and there was a pattern to them. And the implication was that, if I had learnt it, then I could *unlearn* it by changing the pattern that created it.

Other questions Nigel would ask would have the effect of opening up a new way of seeing something that was immensely liberating and in those moments I would have the feeling that burdens I had been carrying for years had been dropped, leaving me free to connect with some of my deepest hopes. Typically, these questions focused on the rules and injunctions I carried around in my head – the 'must do this' and 'have to do that' or 'got to do it this way' statements I took for granted. What I learnt was that most of these rules were either complete exaggerations or just plain nonsense that I had taken over from other people! Learning to make up my own rules and to remain true to them was the key to becoming emotionally healthy again.

By the time I had ended therapy (it took a year) I was fixed on one thing: I wanted to do some of the things Nigel made look so easy. I wanted to learn enough about human beings so that I, too, could know exactly where to look for the root of an emotional problem. And then I would know which questions to ask! I did not know then that a skill like this takes years to develop. I am still learning as I write this!

My first port of call (we are now up to 1988) was to take a training course in Ericksonian hypnosis and therapy. I had been intrigued by Milton Erickson when I was in a bookstore one day looking for more to read on therapy so that I could understand what Nigel was doing to my head. I had seen a complete shelf of books on 'Milton Erickson' and, when I browsed in them, I was struck by the simplicity and strangeness of his work as well as its emotional depth. A man with chronic headaches who prided himself on his honesty was cured by advising him that his headaches were there because he was being dishonest about his difficulties with his wife and children, and it was time he did something about it. A woman with depression, which followed a long history of abuse and rejection from her parents, was taught to reconnect to her anger over her treatment, accept her 'shocking' emotions, and also her right to build a life on her own terms. Another woman with a stomach ulcer was cured after Erickson heard her say that she couldn't 'stomach' her bullying sister. Her ulcer cleared up after she told her sister to stop calling her up on the phone every day with unwanted 'advice'.

I picked these examples because they illustrate one of the principles I learnt from Erickson and which is a key part of the Reverse Therapy approach. And that is the importance of understanding what symptoms are doing in our lives before we try to change them, much less resist them. Making a connection between symptoms and the situations that triggered them led first to emotional insight, then to acceptance of the purpose of the symptoms, and then on to uncovering what needed to be done in order to abolish the body's need to produce symptoms in the first place.

There is much more to Erickson's work than this but I am only referring to that part of it which bears directly on Reverse Therapy and the underlying theme of this book, which is to work with Bodymind to understand and resolve symptoms.

What Milton Erickson taught me

One of the most important aspects of Erickson's work was his emphasis on unconscious communication. Erickson believed in the Unconscious Mind – I no longer do so because I believe that most of what we think is produced by the 'Unconscious' is actually the work of Bodymind (I will explain this in more detail later). Erickson thought that the Unconscious Mind had important reasons for producing symptoms – reasons that had to do with protecting the Self from harm. For example, he once worked with a woman with chronic Eczema. This is a disabling skin condition that causes severe itching and rashes. The woman had a troubled life with many stressors, mostly involving family conflict. Erickson listened to her descriptions of her troubled family life for a long time before observing, in a very suggestive way:

> *'It seems to me that you have a lot of emotions and a little Eczema...'*

This comment was probably delivered in an intensely suggestive way so that the client was invited to pay attention to the unconscious reasons her Bodymind had for producing her Eczema. The client actually became quite angry when Erickson said this and in fact walked out of his office. Notice that in doing so she is already falling in line with what Erickson had pointed out *('...you have a lot of emotions... ')* and is setting herself up for the cure. She called him a week later and, sure enough, her symptoms had abated. The more emotions she had, the less her Bodymind needed to produce symptoms to tell her that it was time she accepted her emotions and acted on them. Walking out on Erickson was one way she acted on that message; speaking up to her family was another. In that way the original emotion was released, and so was the symptom pattern that created the Eczema.

Erickson's work has been extremely influential since he died in 1980 and the people who studied with him have often gone on to establish new forms of therapy. Reverse Therapy owes much to Erickson, in particular the insight that all symptoms have a meaning and a purpose and that healing comes about when we uncover that purpose.

The ideas of Dr Ernest Rossi

One of Erickson's pupils – and co-writer of several books with him – was Dr Ernest Rossi who developed many new ideas from Erickson's work and made important links to Psychobiology – which is the study of Bodymind communication.

In his ground-breaking work The Psychobiology of Mind-Body Healing, Dr Rossi has shown that symptoms arise when Bodymind remembers difficult experiences and stores the information away in the Emotional brain as a chemical memory. Whenever similar experiences come up the chemical memory is activated and chemical messengers are used to tell the body how to respond. Thus different parts of Bodymind are in communication with each other – the Emotional Brain, the glands, the skin, muscles, gut and Immune system and so on. And Bodymind is also in communication with *us* – using the symptoms as 'codes' to flag up that we are back in a difficult situation and need to learn how to do something about it.

All this will be explained in more detail later in this book but for now I just want to put on record that Reverse Therapy is indebted to Dr Rossi's work. For at the time when I was still struggling to understand the relationship between the Mind and the Brain and to work out how therapy could help people recover from physical problems, he was one of the first to show that the body has an intelligence of its own and that this intelligence is centred on the Emotional Brain.

Therapy can help people free themselves from symptoms when we tap into the 'chemical memory' (Rossi calls this 'State-dependent memory') used by Bodymind to create warning signals about situations. When we find out what Bodymind has learned about these situations, and why they are a problem, we are in a position to help clients learn how to do something different. When the client has overcome the difficulty, Bodymind picks up that there is no longer a problem and it dissolves the chemical memory. When that happens the symptoms go with it.

The final piece in the jigsaw: symptom communication

We come now to the last piece in the jigsaw of what eventually became Reverse Therapy. By 1999 I was still largely using hypnosis to explore symptom states and help my clients understand the deeper meaning of their symptoms. After that time I realised that trance was not necessary for people to do this. In fact the rigmarole that usually goes with hypnosis often got in the way. People would be so intent on listening to my suggestions and working up a trance state that they had little attention left over for working through the symptom. Besides, there were far simpler methods that meant that clients could do it for themselves. For example, in the Focusing work pioneered by Eugene Gendlin, clients simply tune in to the sensations that arise in their personal Bodymind when they have emotions and symptoms. They then go through a process of simply 'asking' the symptom state (the 'chemical memory') questions like:

- 'What do you want for me?'
- 'Why is it important for you to be in my life?'
- 'What can I learn from you?'
- 'What would you like me to do now?'

Answers to questions like these make it easier to construct what we call a 'symptom-message' and put it into words. We then get a simple statement which sums up what it is that Bodymind feels is the problem and what Bodymind wants the client to do about it.

For example, in the case described in the box on the next page, Peter's symptom-message was:

'My symptoms are here to tell me not to swallow any more unfair demands from others and speak up for my own needs now'.

Although Gendlin (and other innovators like Rossi himself, Fritz Perls and Steve Gilligan, to name a few) showed me a way to access the symptom-message more directly, we don't use questions like these in Reverse therapy any more. This is because most people are unused to working with Bodymind and may find it difficult to 'talk' to their symptoms and answer the questions.

An early case

In the early days, when I was still experimenting with these ideas, I worked with a male client who had suffered from Irritable Bowel Syndrome for nine years.

The symptoms were bloating, abdominal pain, diarrhoea and nausea. Peter was vaguely aware that his condition became worse if he experienced worries over his family or his work as a lawyer.

He was advised that his symptoms were the complex result of interactions between his mind, his body, his emotions and his environment. When he assented to this he was asked to focus on the sensations of discomfort in his gut and it was suggested that those sensations contained an important message about his problem and soon he would know more about it. He was asked to remember a time when the symptoms were particularly strong and pay attention to any feelings, images and thoughts that came up that would contain clues to 'the message'. After a while, a surprised look came over his face but he was left in peace to 'digest' the message.

When he came to he commented that he had had a shock. An image of a gag came up and he clearly got the idea that his symptoms appeared when he could no longer 'swallow' any more demands from other people. After that we did some practical work on speaking up more firmly to people who imposed on him. Satisfied that he now had some new strategies that would help him deal with the problem, he went 'back inside' and 'asked' his symptom if it was happy with his solutions. Immediately his discomfort subsided. His symptoms quickly cleared up as he became more and more disciplined in dealing with demands from other people. Soon, he was entirely free of symptoms.

In Reverse therapy we work in a fundamentally different way, by taking the client back to life events in which the symptoms first appeared and looking at the environmental pressures they were going through at the time. We ask them to recall the feelings, sensations, emotions and symptoms that were coming up at the time and get a sense of what it was their Bodymind was trying to tell them through the symptoms. There are three other main differences between the Reverse Therapy approach and other methods. The first is that some of the other approaches don't actually develop a symptom-message; they merely try to understand what the symptom is doing there. In my view this is not enough because Bodymind requires action to resolve the problem so that it doesn't need to send symptoms any more in order to protect and guide the individual. Another main difference is that in some hands the idea is to get rid of the symptom as quickly as possible. We treat symptoms as helpful messages that need to be understood first before they can go away – and they will certainly not go away until the client has learned to abide by their advice. The final difference is that we teach our clients how body intelligence actually works through the Emotional Brain and the glands to create the symptoms. More will be said about this in later chapters but the key point here is that knowing what is happening in the body when symptoms come up dispels fear of them and gives the client more control over them.

Reverse therapy can be – and is – used to resolve many conditions treated by traditional psychotherapy, such as Anxiety, Depression and other emotional disorders, as well as symptomatic conditions such as Irritable Bowel Syndrome, Eczema, Insomnia and certain types of Auto-immune disease. However, the focus of this book is on the treatment for Chronic Fatigue Syndrome/M.E. and Fibromyalgia as these are the conditions for which Reverse Therapy is mainly used in the UK. In a later book I will describe how Reverse therapy can work with other problems.

I first began teaching other professionals these ideas in 1999 although at that time I had not yet come up with the name 'Reverse therapy'. In March 2002 I offered an up-to-date version of this approach in a new seminar, with many additions and revisions to my work. During the summer of 2002 one of my students on that course, Dr David Mickel, experimented with the ideas I had taught him and found that they could also be applied to M.E., Chronic Fatigue Syndrome and Fibromyalgia cases. We worked together for eighteen months on this new service, at which point I finally came up with the name 'Reverse therapy' for this new approach in October 2002.

After this collaboration had run its natural course, I decided to set up Reverse Therapy UK in the summer of 2004. The main reason for this is to ensure the training and supervision of Reverse therapists in the United Kingdom on the basis of clearly defined professional and ethical standards. Our higher aim is to offer Reverse Therapy to Chronic Fatigue Syndrome/M.E. and Fibromyalgia sufferers throughout the world. If you have this book in your hands you can be sure that you are in the forefront of a new revolution in Bodymind healing as many more readers discover the powerful tools that we have to offer.

Chapter 2

From Headstuff to Bodymind

In this chapter you will learn:

> ➤ *The difference between Headmind and Bodymind*
> ➤ *About the emotional intelligence of Bodymind*
> ➤ *How Headmind is based on other people's rules*
> ➤ *Why Headmind tricks can damage your health*
> ➤ *How Bodymind uses feelings, emotions and symptoms to communicate to you*

Why Headmind is over-rated

The key to understanding Reverse therapy lies in understanding the importance of Bodymind. At the same time this entails a revision of what we mean by Mind and discarding the old practice of assigning Intelligence purely to 'the Head'.

Headmind refers to the kind of thinking that gets taught in schools and colleges and universities. In different ways it forms the basis for understanding language, mathematics, history and science. The skills required include remembering things by rote, putting things into words, learning rules, deducing and analysing things, conceptualising, explaining and arguing. Headmind also includes imagination, which we can use creatively to predict the future, come up with new solutions or construct works of art. Purely intellectual definitions of Mind are heavily over-emphasised in western cultures and, as we shall see below, can be a source of illness.

Over the past twenty years or so, researchers have pointed to the fact that human beings exhibit many different kinds of intelligence, not just the ones that get tested by intelligence tests or school examinations. These include musical intelligence, artistic intelligence, athletic intelligence and emotional intelligence. To understand and work with Bodymind requires a particular type of

16

emotional intelligence, as described in the next paragraph.

In a previous book I co-wrote with my friend, Roy Johnson, entitled *Communicating with Emotional Intelligence*, we asserted that Emotional Intelligence consists of Interpersonal skills and Intrapersonal skills. *Interpersonal* skills belong to socially adept people; individuals who are able to 'read' other people well, empathising with their feelings, motives and needs, and adapting what they say and do accordingly. These are the great therapists, communicators and relationship-builders. All Reverse therapists are trained to develop these skills.

Intrapersonal skills, on the other hand, relate more specifically to personal Bodymind work. They are based on the ability to detect, understand and act upon one's *own* moods, feelings, emotions and needs. And, as we shall see, emotionally intelligent people are also able to notice when they are coming down with the first, faint symptoms of distress and take appropriate, corrective action. One of the primary goals of Reverse therapy is to foster this skill in our clients.

Headmind, on its own, cannot help people become emotionally intelligent. In fact it often gets in the way by interrupting, de-pressing and explaining away our emotions. Let's look at examples of all three of these processes in action:

- Interrupting. We get into conversation with someone who seems plausible and charming but inwardly we experience a feeling of unease. This is our Bodymind telling us, using its finely attuned store of emotional memories, that the person is not to be trusted. But Headmind interrupts this feeling and directs us to be polite, sociable and friendly.

- De-pressing. We are stuck in a dead-end job or a relationship that is going nowhere. We feel sad and alone. This is Bodymind warning us that we need to take action to re-ignite our relationship with the employer or the partnership, or move on. But Headmind denies this emotion because it fears taking a risk. So we 'de-press' our scary emotions and lose the capacity to feel and, with it, our

17

passion for life. Instead of relating to the emotion of sadness we have suppressed it, although it still remains in the Bodymind system, waiting to be expressed and understood.

- Explaining away. A child is rude, abusive or inconsiderate. Inwardly we feel angry or frustrated. But Headmind thinks we are not being a 'good parent' if we express that emotion and triggers off a process in which we reason: 'she's having a hard time at school' or 'he's going through that adolescent phase' or even 'they're good children really'.

Unhealthy Headmind does this because, in reality, it is created by conditioning. It is filled with the assumptions, rules and ideas of the society we were born into and which we have internalised, so much so that we actually come to believe that these assumptions, rules and ideas are our own. It aims at conformity and 'being reasonable'. It avoids risk and thereby creates fear. Through programming, it wants us to be 'good children', work hard, stay out of trouble and shoulder any burdens that come our way without complaint, even if they are unbearable. It never, never wishes us to be authentic. Instead it wants us to follow the crowd and fosters dependency on other people. It distrusts the 'irrational' messages from Bodymind and tries to resist them. Should Bodymind respond by intensifying emotions (as can often happen prior to illness) it assumes that something 'weird' must be happening and seeks the attention of a medical doctor or a psychotherapist.

Sadly, this wrong work of Headmind may actually lead us to ignore our distress on the assumption that 'others come first' and that we are letting people down if we admit that something is wrong. After years of this kind of denial we may settle down to a life of cynical resignation in which illness and unhappiness are accepted as natural and inevitable – the 'way things are'. People who point out a better way, based on spiritual or emotional awareness and personal autonomy, may be dismissed as 'weird' or unrealistic.

How can we detect when Unhealthy forms of Headmind have taken over? There are numerous clues, some of which have already been mentioned while others are listed below:

- Thinking we must be 'selfish' if we focus on having our own emotional needs met.
- Blaming others for our problems or distress ('If it wasn't for you...').
- Rigidly adhering to the rules set by others without questioning them ('That's what the boss says and that must be right...').
- Constantly saying 'I must...', 'I should...' or 'I have to...' in everyday talk.
- Abusing food, drugs and alcohol instead of attending to our emotional needs.
- Remaining victims instead of taking responsibility and speaking up for ourselves.
- Blindly following other people's explanations and prescriptions for health and happiness.
- Manipulating others (including therapists) so that we can avoid the hard work of listening to Bodymind and becoming healthy .

Unhealthy environments create unhealthy minds. These may include schools, homes and offices but, most importantly, unhealthy thinking is transmitted by unhealthy people, many of whom have themselves been taught to belittle or disregard their emotions. How many of us, as children, were told when we were sad that 'you'll get over it', that when we expressed joy that we must not get 'over-excited', that only 'wimps' cried, or that our anger at hurt or injustice was 'childish'. Unless we were lucky enough to be surrounded by warm and emotionally intelligent people we gradually learned to assume that emotional deadness was normal and that an inability to remain detached from our emotions was a sign of illness. This may explain the ever-increasing prescriptions of drugs like anti-depressants and Ritalin (which dampens mood in so-called 'Hyperactive' children). In fact, as we shall see, Bodymind is essentially child-like and not childish. And Emotional Intelligence depends on our capacity for innocent perception, acceptance of our own emotional truth, and permission to express those same truths. But first we have to ignore Headmind and give ourselves permission to do this.

All about 'Bananas'

One of the most common traps created by Headmind are what I call 'bananas'. A banana is something Headmind tells us we have to have to hang on to even when trying to hang on to it brings us nothing but misery and illness. It is a kind of fixation in which we imagine we have to try and live up to somebody else's standards – 'lovable', 'successful', 'obedient', etc. In my view the bananas many people live by are one of the prime reasons for unhappiness and, if left undetected, can lead to illness, as I shall explain later.

When we come across bananas in Reverse Therapy we often tell clients the following story to explain the idea of a banana:

In some parts of Africa they still use a traditional way to catch a monkey. The hunter will make a small wicker basket, with bars wide enough apart for a monkey's paw. Then he will find a grove where the monkeys live and put it on the ground with a banana inside. Then the hunter hides up a tree. Sooner or later a monkey will come along and inspect the basket. Finding the banana the monkey grasps it and holds on tight. But the bars aren't wide enough for it to withdraw its hand while holding a banana. So it waits. And waits. It is still waiting when the hunter throws a net over it and hauls it off to the market.

We know a monkey's brain is only a little smaller than that of a human. You would think it was smart enough to let go of the banana. The reason it doesn't is not because it is stupid but because its demand for the banana is stronger than any instinct for survival. The same principle applies to human beings. All of us have 'bananas' we hold on to for dear life, even when holding on is against our best interests. One thing that stops people changing is fear of what will happen to them if they let go of the banana.

Here are some common bananas:

- I must be loved.
- I have to be successful.
- I must have more money.
- I must not show anger.

- I should always be a good parent.
- I must be a good boy/girl.
- I must not rock the boat.
- I have to help people.
- I must not be selfish.
- I must have revenge.

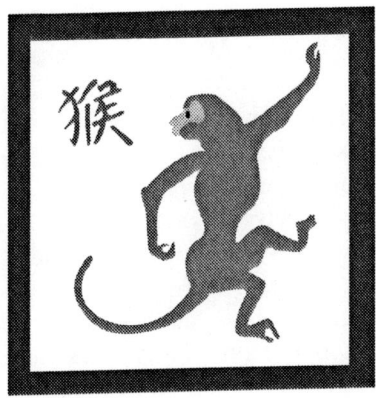

Holding on to any of these bananas is hard work and can lead to physical exhaustion! Until we learn to let go we may have to go through a draining routine of trying to please others, taking on ever more overtime in order to earn that bonus, putting up with abuse, taking on other people's burdens and swallowing our own frustration when all this gets too much for us. In some cases, when we realise that our efforts earn us no thanks or gratitude, we might become resentful. Losing sight of the fact that no one ever asked us to hold on to the banana, we start to blame others and, even to try and get revenge through hurtful words and behaviour. Now we have added conflict with others to the list of environmental pressures that we have to cope with.

Notice that these banana statements all contain the words 'must', 'should' or 'have to'. There is nothing in itself wrong with wanting to be a good parent, making money or wanting to be loved. But there will always be times when we make mistakes, suffer financial loss or lose the affection of a partner. And if we cannot accept that sometimes we are not good parents, that we won't have much money, or that we may have to be single for a while, then we are in trouble. We will worry about things, trying ever harder to get back what it is we can't do without, rather like a junkie hurrying around trying to get his next fix. We end by overloading ourselves with burdens – giving in to our children's tantrums, working ten hours a day, or putting up with an abusive partner in order not to be alone. The more we try and hold on to the banana the more we lose touch with ourselves and our deepest emotional needs. Worst of all we end up feeling trapped, helpless and the victim of circumstances.

How do we release a banana? The first step is to realise we have one. This can be difficult as we often see our own bananas as 'necessities' that we can't do without. If they are pointed out to us we may say things like 'But *everybody* wants more money!' or 'That's just the way I am – I can't say "no" to someone who needs me.' To many people their bananas are part of an unchangeable reality – just 'the way things are'. They miss the fact that, under the influence of other people's rules, and conditioning, they have turned desirable qualities into obsessions. It is natural to want to be helpful and kind, to do our best in our work, to make the best of our talents and to make enough money to support those we love. But when these wishes become all-or-nothing fixations in which we never give ourselves time to nurture ourselves then the cage traps us.

The simplest way out of the trap is to do the direct opposite of whatever we were doing while we were still holding the banana. Instead of working more, we work less. Instead of seeking revenge, we ask for reconciliation. Instead of repressing our anger we find a way to express it constructively. All these moves require that we take a risk and give up the habits of a lifetime. Many people find this difficult, scary and even strange at first. They may also have to be firm in dealing with people who have long been used to the way they were. But the emotional benefits are enormous and so is the eventual impact on their health.

In Reverse Therapy we encourage clients to reconnect to their Bodymind needs and learn to deal more effectively with environmental pressures. There are two main types of pressure. The first are the demands that are imposed on us by other people and situations. These include young people facing school and college exams; parents bringing up children; families coping with illness, poverty and deprivation; employees with demanding jobs and employers; employers with the stresses of running a business; partners who are in conflict, or who are going through separation and divorce; people who are isolated from the community; survivors of emotional, sexual and physical abuse; children looking after elderly parents, and so on. All these situations impose different types of challenge and require different responses if the person is to remain in balance and stay healthy.

The second type of pressure also comes from the environment but in a subtly different way. These are the pressures that come from unhealthy work of Headmind and which we took over from other people. Through conditioning we may have learnt that we had to deny or explain away our emotions. In fact, if we were brought up in a western culture we probably learned that Bodymind was of little importance and should be ignored. That if we suffered from symptoms of distress we should go and see a doctor so that they could be suppressed with the aid of drugs. Through following the example of others we may have internalised a banana that dictated we should work too hard or try to be 'perfect' children, partners and parents.

In fact both types of environmental pressure often work in tandem with one another. We come up against a trial or a crisis that requires adaptation and change. This may mean giving up or scaling down other commitments, getting help, making time and space for ourselves or making it clear to others that there are limits to what we can do. If we have been programmed not to do any of these things then adaptation becomes very difficult. We may become frightened, driven, helpless and scared. We feel unable to cope but don't want it to look as if we are letting others down. The next step is a state of 'dis-ease' (see next chapter) in which we are out of sync with ourselves. Inevitably, we develop distressing emotions and symptoms of illness as Bodymind wakes up and tries to warn us about the predicament we are in.

Fortunately, Bodymind is not easily deterred from its task of mobilising the body to deal with the emergency and it makes powerful attempts to remind us of our duty to ourselves.

The wisdom of Bodymind

We defined Bodymind earlier as the intelligence of the body. It is in fact an organising intelligence that brings together several functions:

The Two Zen Monks

This is an old story that perfectly illustrates how bananas work.

Two Zen Monks were on a pilgrimage to another monastery. They had both taken strict vows not to touch other people and to remain silent at all times.

After many days they came to a river. On the bank was a beautiful young peasant girl who could not get across because the water was too deep. She asked the Monks if one of them would carry her across.

The first Monk said, 'All right', carried her across on his back, set her down, and wished her a safe journey.

The two Monks continued on their route but the second Monk brooded. After another two days of walking he could no longer contain himself and burst out,

'Why did you do that? It is a disgrace! You know we are not allowed to touch or speak to anyone!'

'Let it go,' said the first Monk, 'you're still carrying her'.

- Emotional recall of experiences from the past.
- Computer-like processing of sensory information.

24

- Matching present experiences to responses used in the past using 'emotional radar'
- Super-fast activation of the glands and other message-stations.
- Arousal of the body's natural defence mechanisms against threat.

The wisdom of Bodymind consists in picking up information about the experiences we are having and developing a prepared response, or, if one is not available, then indicating that a new response needs to be learnt. To take some simple examples: if you are a good tennis player then when you get on the court you are probably going to be pleasantly excited about the game as Bodymind keys you up to the right pitch of arousal. As the game starts you comfortably get into gear and automatically you use all the strokes you have learnt from the other games you have played in.

By contrast, you are in a foreign country and don't know the language well. You ask for directions to the beach but no one understands your accent. As frustration increases, your voice gets louder and louder while you repeat the word for 'beach' and you may even flip back into English. That frustration is Bodymind's way of telling you that you need to slow down and spend more time practicing your accent. Just as your exhilaration on the tennis court was Bodymind's way of recalling you to your confidence and skill.

Bodymind communicates to us every day of our lives. It does this through feelings of all kinds, the feeling complexes we label as emotions – these include fear, anger, sadness and disgust – and also through symptoms. In doing so it draws our attention to things and guides us towards action by providing us we a 'feel' for how thing are. It continually acts like our guardian angel, alerting us to when we have a problem, and encouraging us to act when we feel we know what to do next.

Let us take some more examples from everyday life, this time focusing specifically on feelings, emotions and symptoms. Bear in mind when looking at each example that Bodymind is using changes in body chemistry to communicate to us in every case.

Feelings

- You are walking alone at night along an empty street. The hairs on your neck begin to prick up when you notice that someone is following behind. Bodymind wishes you to be alert, move more quickly and head for a place of safety.

- You are having a hard day at work. There is too much to do and you are already behind on schedule on a number of projects. Then you get a phone call from the boss who tells you that a customer has complained and you will have to drop everything and deal with it. You experience a sinking, heavy sensation around the heart. Bodymind wishes you to have a frank conversation with your boss.

- You are a working parent with three young children and your partner is ill in hospital after an accident. There are numerous financial worries and you are struggling to look after the children, maintain the home and pay the bills. Each night as you get into bed you experience a buzzing sensation in the head as your mind races over your worries. Bodymind is urging you to get more support from other people.

Emotions

- After months of turmoil your partner finally tells you that he or she is ending the relationship. You experience a great sadness accompanied by tears, a heavy sensation in the chest and back, and a tightness in the throat. Bodymind is alerting you to your loss, get other sources of emotional support and get ready to move on to better things.

- A person you have long distrusted, and who has behaved badly to you in the past, proves true to form and slanders you behind your back. When a friend tells you what has happened you experience disgust. Your facial muscles crease, your stomach heaves slightly and you swallow involuntarily. Bodymind wishes you to do what you can to protect and distance yourself from this person.

26

- You are waiting at home for your child to come back from school. He is over an hour late and you know the school bus has come and gone. You try his mobile phone and it is switched off. You experience a sudden fear. Your breathing is shallow, your chest and stomach muscles clench and you feel slightly nauseous. Bodymind wishes you to go out and look for your child.

Symptoms

- You have been sitting at the computer most of the day trying to finish an article in time for the last post. At the same time the phone has rung constantly, friends have dropped in uninvited and now your teenage daughter throws a tantrum when you refuse to drive her to a friend's house ten minutes' walk away. You develop a splitting headache. Bodymind urgently requires you to take some time out for yourself! It may also be warning you that you have a banana about having to be 'nice'.

- The business you have spent years developing is now failing. Orders have dried up, your creditors are taking advantage of your situation and are paying late and you get daily phone calls from your bank manager ordering you to reduce the overdraft. Every night you go to sleep and wake up at three in the morning completely awake. No matter how hard you try you cannot get more than four hours sleep at night. By mid-day you are exhausted. Bodymind wishes you to get some professional and personal help immediately. It may also be warning you that you have a banana about having to do everything all by yourself.

- You are looking after your elderly parents as well as your own family. They live miles away and it is a four-hour trip there and back. They are frail and increasingly demanding. They show little gratitude for your efforts to care for them and complain incessantly as soon as you arrive. They also demand that you visit them every day. You refuse but they will not let the subject drop. They go on and on about what a terrible daughter you are and how they prefer your brother

27

(who never visits them). They remind you about all they have done for you and drag up old grievances about you, your husband and your children. Over time the skin rash you used to have years ago as a child returns and soon your skin is covered with itching, red sores. Bodymind wishes you to start setting some boundaries between you and your parents and to get ready to speak up. It may also be warning you that you have a banana about having to be a perfect daughter.

In some cases, especially with simple feeling reactions, Bodymind attempts to alert us to an area of concern and to let us know that our interests are threatened. Perhaps the most striking example of this is the way in which a mother will awake with a sudden shock in the middle of the night and realise that her baby is crying. Consciously, she was deeply asleep and yet, throughout, Bodymind continued to monitor her environment in case anything untoward might be happening. It then utilised an alarm mechanism stored in the Emotional Brain to produce the mild shock that woke her up. We will say more about this mechanism later.

In general, Bodymind produces feeling states, emotions and early symptoms in order to alert us to the fact that an event of deep personal concern has come up and that a response is required.

We then develop a 'feel' for the situation and, if Headmind is working properly, we soon work out what to do, the emotion is worked out and Bodymind extinguishes the emotion and goes back on standby. If Headmind is not working properly and we try to deny or 'de-press' the emotion then no action is taken, emotional expression is blocked and Bodymind turns to other ways of adapting and drawing our attention to the problem.

As a rule, when we are under stress, Bodymind progresses from vague feelings of unease, to more clearly defined, and longer-lasting, emotions, to mild symptoms of illness and then on to chronic symptoms. Thus the symptoms get 'louder and louder'. Sadly, in some cases, such as cancer, if early-stage symptoms are not picked up and acted upon, major symptoms may set in and can prove irreversible.

28

The case of Elliott

A real-life case that occurred many years ago shows clearly what happens if we are unable to connect to Bodymind and be guided by feelings and emotions.

An operation to remove a tumour from Elliott's brain had caused a loss of healthy tissue, which meant the connection between the Thinking centres and the Emotional Brain had been severed. The result was that Elliott was unable to feel any emotions. If shown gory photographs of crash victims, Elliott reacted as if he were looking at something rather boring. Lacking an access to his own feelings Elliott was unable to make decisions the rest of us would take for granted – like whether it was time to get up in the morning or meet up with a friend. In fact he had not the slightest interest in things that happened to him, even when they were disastrous. He saw no particular reason why he should do a job well (although he could understand – in theory – how and why it should be done). Nor did he have the emotional staying power to see a job through to the end. He made a number of bad decisions – based on his inability to 'read' other people's motives – which led to eventually to personal and business failure.

Without Bodymind to help him develop a feel for the right thing to do he was helpless.

The analogy we use for this progression from feelings to symptoms in Reverse Therapy is that of the 'messenger at the door'. Imagine you have a message to deliver to a friend that is of vital importance to her safety. Like Bodymind in its relationship with the Self, you want to help your friend and you will do whatever it takes to protect her. You go to your friend's house and you can see the lights are on and that she is at home. You knock gently on the door and wait but there is no answer. You knock louder and still there is no answer, so you try the bell. You can hear someone moving around inside so you knock still more loudly hoping that she will open the door. Your 'symptom noises' are still not getting any response so in sheer frustration you end up banging on the door and shouting up to the window…

As soon as we 'open the door' to Bodymind and listen to the message that it wishes to convey to us through the symptoms, and act accordingly, then Bodymind has no further need to use symptoms to communicate to us. The mechanisms in the Emotional Brain that are used to create symptoms are switched off and Bodymind goes back on standby, continuing to monitor the environment until some other issue comes up that requires our attention.

In general, Bodymind strives towards:

- Equilibrium – a balance between what we do for others and what we do for ourselves.
- Authenticity – the expression of our emotional truth.
- Personal satisfaction and fulfilment.
- Excitement, interest, deep curiosity.
- Engagement in mutually rewarding relationships with other people.
- Happiness, joy, serenity and inner peace.
- Building environments (homes, families, work) which foster emotional well-being and health.

When Headmind is working properly it helps Bodymind maintain health by:

- Staying in the present and noticing what is actually going on
- Setting realistic limits to what one can and what one cannot do
- Making decisions and planning for action
- Putting things into words and speaking up
- Drawing boundaries between self and others
- Recognising bananas and letting them go
- Is simple, direct, honest and self-respectful
- Learns how to say 'no' to unrealistic demands from others
- Looks for new solutions to old problems
- 'Goes with the flow' and adapts as situations and people change
- Sees the humour in situations

All these are qualities that Reverse Therapists foster and encourage in our clients. We also help them to understand that there is a natural cycle in Bodymind communication that leads from recognition of an emotion (or a symptom) through consideration, decision and action to closure. Following this discipline spontaneously allows Bodymind to switch off the mechanisms that produce emotions and symptoms and return to standby mode. This is illustrated in the Flowchart shown on the next page.

What this flowchart illustrates is that there is a natural progression from encountering an event, emotionally evaluating it, and then using Headmind to take action, based on the emotion given, to 'close out' the transaction and extinguish the emotion. This is the healthy cycle that leads to positive feelings of pleasure at getting something done. The unhealthy cycle will lead to blocks, frustration and increased emotional signals from Bodymind that we experience negatively.

Here are three of the most commonly cycled emotions, along with some comments on what it is Bodymind generally wishes us to do in each case:

Flowchart of Bodymind communication

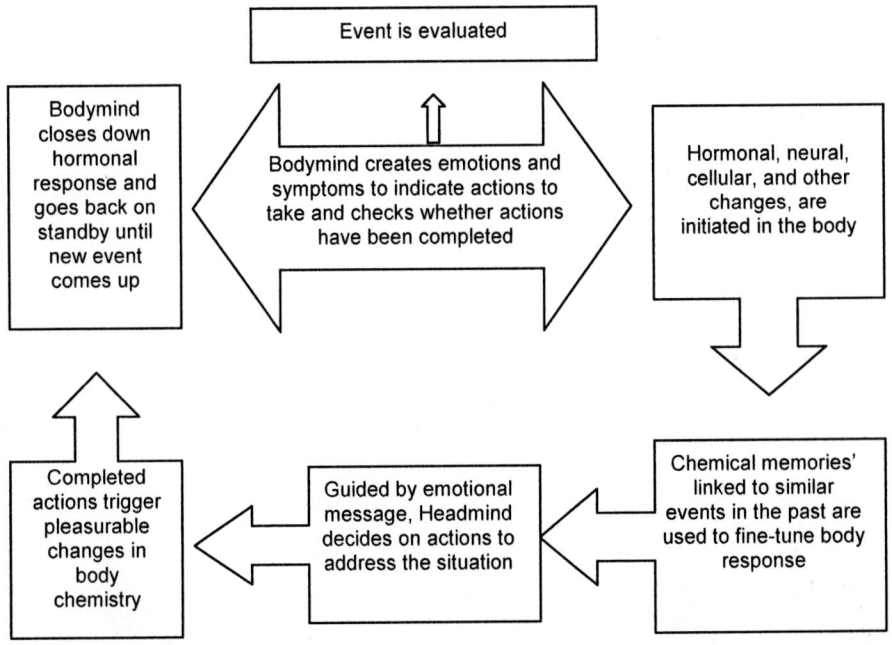

Fear. In normal conditions this emotion tells us that we (or someone close to us) is unsafe in some way. This may be because we/they are actually in danger and we need to move out of the way quickly. Another reason we experience fear is because Bodymind picks up that we are low in confidence. This may be because we have undergone experiences (such as illness) that left us feeling helpless. Or it may be because we haven't yet learned to master something, such as learning to ride a bike when we were children and kept falling off.

If Headmind blocks action because it has been programmed not to take risks then Bodymind intensifies the Fear response to let us know that the problem has not been resolved. In most cases the correct response is to take small steps towards mastery of the problem, getting some help along the way if we can, and gradually raising confidence. This is what most of us did when we learned to rise a bike. We did not simply give up learning – we just took more care when we next got back on!

Anger. In normal conditions this tells us that some other person has deliberately violated our rights. Bodymind wishes us to restore the situation by speaking up for ourselves and making it clear that the violation should not be repeated. Alternatively, the anger may follow a longer series of frustrations in which we allowed others to take liberties. Again, what is called for is a restoration of our rights. In abnormal conditions we may be holding a banana that dictates that other people should always do what we want and that they must be 'evil' if they don't. In this case it would be best to become less dependent on other people and learn to do more for ourselves.

If Headmind blocks action because it has been programmed not to 'make a fuss' then Bodymind again turns up the emotion and we may be left for months – or even years – with a seething, inner resentment, continually replaying the injustice over and over in Headmind. William Blake's poem 'A Poison Tree' springs to mind here:

> I was angry with my friend:
> I told my wrath, my wrath did end.
> I was angry with my foe:

I told it not, my wrath did grow.

Blake goes on to describe how the wrath continued to grow, 'watered in tears' and 'sunned' with false smiles until it turned into a poisonous apple. At last the foe ate it and was found dead beside the tree. But it is unlikely that the narrator was emotionally healthier for that. If anger has been allowed to go for too long then, if we have not taken the opportunity to speak up and resolve the matter, then it is better to forgive.

Shame. This very natural emotion is linked to remorse. It tells us we have done something wrong and need to make amends. It carries the feeling that we have let ourselves down and have lost self-respect.

Bodymind wishes us to do what we can to repair the harm we have done and, if that is impossible, then exercise charity in some other way. We may also need to go through a process of self-forgiveness prior to moving on.

If Headmind blocks action because it is afraid of the consequences of owning up, then the shame turns into guilt – we are ashamed of what we have done but are frightened of being found out. If Headmind is programmed to assume that we must always be right, and never wrong, then no action is taken but the feeling remains, this time turning into fear of judgment, which we may try to cover over with self-righteousness.

Notice that, in every case, there is a positive, natural expression of emotion which leads to appropriate action, thus closing the cycle (see Flowchart). There is also a negative expression of emotion which comes about when it is blocked or poisoned by wrong work of Headmind – interrupting, de-pressing, explaining things away or holding on to bananas.

If action is blocked then Bodymind actually does something rather interesting – it evaluates the avoidance of action as a *new problem*. It notices that something has *not* been done, re-evaluates the situation and then creates new emotions in order to get our attention

33

and encourage us to get to work. Bodymind never gives up until it feels the problem is resolved.

Ann's case 1

Ann came to see me after suffering from Fibromyalgia symptoms for eight years. My first impression was that she looked absolutely exhausted, as indeed she was. She also reported severe muscle and joint pain over most of her body, sleep disturbance, fatigue, headaches, and vertigo.

Reverse Therapy always starts by taking a careful case history, focusing particularly on life-events that were occurring just before symptoms first appeared.

In Ann's case there were three significant events. One was her mother's death, the second was a conflict with her sister, and the third was continuing bullying from her in-laws. First symptoms occurred the week after her mother's funeral.

Ann was very upset by the death of her mother, whom she considered her most important source of support and her best friend. She was shocked and upset by the fact that her sister took away, without permission, all her mother's jewellery and tried to take possession of her house. From respect for her mother, and because she was frightened of her sister she said nothing. Her sister did in fact take the house and Ann was still angry about this eleven years later.

Her husband's parents had always treated her badly – either ignoring her or telling her what to do, or complaining to her husband about her 'attitude' until she learned to 'keep her mouth shut'. In fact, they behaved in almost the same intimidating way as her sister. But without support from her husband (who told her he just wanted 'a quiet life') or from her dead mother, she felt unable to cope. *(Conclusion: Chapter 6)*.

Key points to remember:

> *Bodymind is far more intelligent than Headmind and is in tune with our core need for truth, love and personal fulfillment*

> *When Headmind is working properly it carries out the orders of Bodymind*

> *When Headmind is not working properly it tries to take over and to force us to act like everybody else, even when that is not right for us*

> *Bodymind talks to you every day of your life through your feelings, emotions and symptoms*

> *Bodymind only produces symptoms as a last resort when our deepest interests are threatened*

Chapter 3

Bodymind, symptoms and 'dis-ease'

In this chapter you will learn:

- ➤ About 'dis-ease' – the state we get into when Bodymind communication is ignored
- ➤ About the work of Hans Selye
- ➤ How environmental pressures can lead to illness
- ➤ Why the Emotional Brain is the powerhouse of Bodymind
- ➤ How Bodymind uses 'chemical memories' to record what it has learned from experience
- ➤ The crucial role of the Hypothalamus in producing symptoms

How Dis-ease comes about

In the last chapter we looked at Bodymind in general terms. In this chapter we are going to look at how and why Bodymind creates symptoms. On the way we will look at the state of 'dis-ease' that is the condition we fall into when Bodymind is unable to maintain health, thus forcing it to create uncomfortable emotions, and then symptoms, to warn us that we have lost the balance between external pressures and personal needs.

By 'environment' we are not only referring to people and events out there in the real world but also to the internal environment – the rules, regulations and 'bananas' we have taken over from other people and stored away in Headmind. Sometimes Bodymind will strongly disagree with Headmind and may send symptoms to warn us not to listen to it! When this happens it will encourage us to find new ways of dealing with people and situations. For example, if Headmind thinks that it is 'wrong' to ask others for help and we are overwhelmed with work, then Bodymind will signal that we need to do just that! Please bear in mind while you are reading this chapter that Bodymind always focuses on *action and expression* –

physically doing or saying things that solve the problems that come our way. Reverse Therapy does not work by changing Headmind but by bypassing it and focusing on Bodymind.

'Dis-ease', as the hyphen implies, is a state of being in which we are no longer at ease with ourselves. We no longer feel comfortable with our work, our home-life or our relationships with other people. Initially the state of dis-ease comes with uncomfortable feelings or mild distress as Bodymind gently draws our attention to the fact that we are out of balance. Deep down, we may know that something is wrong with our lives but may not be able to put our finger on the problem or, if we do have a idea what it is, we may not know how to put things right.

In the early stages of dis-ease the answer to the problem may be quite simple. It could involve a heart-to-heart talk with a partner, changing the schedule at work, or spending more time on things that are truly important to us. But if problems mount the state of dis-ease becomes more noticeable as Bodymind 'talks' to us more and more urgently. At this point we may become tense and anxious, worried and sleepless, more and more aware that we are becoming over-burdened. We may feel that we never have enough time to do all the things we think we have to do. At this point we may be out of touch with our deepest needs and may even lose the ability to read our own emotions. As the state of dis-ease grows, Headmind becomes increasingly split from Bodymind and stops doing its proper job of putting Bodymind orders into action – identifying solutions, making decisions and taking action. It may even try and take over and block Bodymind altogether – interrupting, depressing, 'explaining' why there is no way out of the trap and belittling symptoms as 'a passing phase' or as something we should see the doctor about.

In the 1930s Hans Selye, a Hungarian psychologist, showed how a state of dis-ease leads to illness. Selye, while still a medical student at the University of Prague, became interested in patients with non-specific illnesses. They often complained of feeling ill although no specific diagnosis could be made. Common symptoms were tiredness, a coated tongue, diffuse aches and pains in the joints, loss of appetite, digestive problems, feverishness, an enlarged spleen or liver, inflamed tonsils, or a skin rash. Only later on would specific illnesses such as liver disease, or Immune system breakdown, become available for medical treatment.

Selye noted that many of these patients had recently been exposed to what he called 'noxious agents' (he later used the term 'stress') by which he meant challenging influences from the environment. In fact he later on established that a considerable number of these patients had been exposed to major life changes in the period just before the appearance of symptoms. Such changes – job loss, death of family members, financial problems, childcare difficulties – required a great deal of adaptation on the part of the individual, which in turn, triggered major changes in body function.

If these life-pressures were not resolved then more chronic problems appeared, such as enlargement of the Adrenal cortex and shrinkage of the Thymus, Spleen and Lymphatic glands as well as pre-ulcerative conditions of the stomach and upper intestine.

Selye saw that the symptoms of non-specific conditions (in which category we also include Chronic Fatigue Syndrome/M.E. and Fibromyalgia) appeared because the individual had failed to adapt to environmental pressures and resolve them. He called this failure to adapt the *General Adaptation Syndrome* (GAS) in which the path from dis-ease to serious illness went through three stages. We will go into more detail on the mechanisms involved later but the general pattern is as follows.

In the First stage, there is a general *Alarm Reaction* in which Bodymind indicates that the state of dis-ease is not being resolved, pressures are getting worse, and the individual is now in trouble. Initially, the Alarm Reaction is a kind of 'wake-up call' in which we are alerted to the growing seriousness of the situation and encouraged to do something about it. Bodymind triggers hormonal changes that put the body on 'red alert' in order to muster energy to deal with the threat and also to use symptoms to let us know that action is required. Emotionally we may experience fear, meaning we need to restore personal safety, or anger, meaning we need to protest about our right to health.

The second stage is the *Resistance* stage. In this phase Bodymind realises that we are not going to do anything about the problem, are ignoring the early-warning symptoms, and resisting the need to change. 'Early-warning' symptoms intensify, partly because the 'red alert' mechanism is stepping up, partly because Bodymind is now using symptoms to indicate that the situation cannot be allowed to continue. Such symptoms may include restlessness, tension, sleep problems, appetite/digestive problems, occasional fatigue and loss of sexual drive. At this stage the symptoms are still quickly reversible once we take action. But if we try to resist the early-stage *symptoms* and 'keep going' – working harder, doing without sleep, giving-in to others' demands, ignoring our need for exercise, intimacy and leisure, and speeding up instead of slowing down – then symptoms become chronic.

In the *Exhaustion* stage, or, as I prefer to call it – the *'Stalemate* stage' Bodymind is still trying to keep the body on 'red alert'. The Adrenal glands, in particular, work ever harder, and in the case of Chronic Fatigue Syndrome/M.E. and Fibromyalgia, they over-stimulate the muscles until they become painful and fatigued, overwork the Gastro-Intestinal tract so that food insensitivities, or nausea, Candida, and an irritable bowel develop, and over-activate the Immune system until it temporarily crashes and is unable to resist viral infections. Some body functions now approach the limit of their ability to keep going under emergency conditions and begin to falter. For example, the Adrenal glands may start to ignore signals from Bodymind to work harder and may decrease their supply of Cortisol to the blood. As we will see later, low Cortisol is a feature of Chronic Fatigue Syndrome /M.E. and Fibromyalgia and, contributes to symptoms of exhaustion, sensitivity to pain, and Immune system dysfunction. At this point the body cannot go on continuing on 'red alert' and Bodymind, realising this, signals ever more frantically for the pressure to be resolved. But stalemate develops because Bodymind is waiting for us to intervene and take action.

Hans Selye's work has been immensely influential. At a time (the 1930s) when it was assumed that all illnesses were caused by either infections, injury, or by genetic defects, he proved that some conditions were produced by problems in adapting to pressure. He

39

was the first to demonstrate the link between environmental problems and the development of symptoms. He also saw that, so long as we fail to adapt and find new ways to deal with those pressures, then the symptoms will escalate through the three stages of Alarm, Resistance and Stalemate.

The key role of the Emotional Brain

It is now time to look more closely at the way in which Bodymind works through the Emotional Brain. Again, it was Hans Selye who first realised that it was this brain system that was responsible for organising the individual's response to environmental pressures. However, in what follows I have also drawn heavily on the work of Dr Ernest Rossi.

The Emotional Brain is located roughly in the middle of the skull, and is at the heart of Bodymind. As the name implies, it creates emotional responses to situations, which in turn guide the rest of the body, and Headmind, towards action. What it actually does is to convert perceptions – sights and sounds – into emotions, providing us with an extremely fast 'emotional opinion' about what is going on around us. The Emotional Brain works so fast that – provided we are attentive to our bodies – we are often aware of our emotions about the situation before we are aware of the situation itself. In Chapter 2, I gave a number of examples of Bodymind in action, but here is a more striking example.

Supposing you are taking a walk in the woods and notice a strange coloured 'stick' in the grass. Let us also suppose for a moment that your Emotional Brain does not work properly and you have to rely on Headmind to help you work things out. Because Headmind works extremely slowly, you stare at the stick for some time and notice that it has some strange, zig-zag marks on it and that it a has a green-brown colouring. You wonder whether some children have been painting sticks in the forest or whether, possibly, someone has lost their flute. You might even start to theorise about ancient, pagan cultures that created the stick as part of their tribal rituals and fantasise that you have made a unique discovery. Suddenly, the 'stick' moves towards you and coils up. Too late, the snake has bitten you. Now compare this with the Emotional Brain response. A split-second before you even became aware of the 'stick' the Emotional Brain has already decided that it is a suspicious object and, bypassing the Thinking Centres, has triggered an immediate 'Alarm' reaction.

The work of Dr. Ryke-Geerd Hamer

One of the most striking confirmations of Selye's discoveries comes out of the work of Dr Ryke-Geerd Hamer over the past twenty years or so. Hamer investigated over 20,000 cancer cases in Germany and wondered why cancer never seems to systematically spread directly from one organ to the surrounding tissue. For example, he never found cancer of the cervix AND cancer of the uterus in the same woman. This suggested that cancer was specific to one particular body function. He also noticed that all his cancer patients seemed to have experienced an emotional conflict prior to onset of their disease, a conflict that had never been fully resolved.

Hamer also came up with some further discoveries. X-rays taken of the skulls of cancer patients showed in all cases a 'dark shadow' somewhere in the brain. These dark spots would be in exactly the same place in the brain for the same types of cancer. There was also a 100% correlation between the dark spot in the brain, the location of the cancer in the body and the specific type of unresolved conflict.

On the basis of these findings, Hamer suggests that when a conflict is not resolved, specific Centres in the brain will malfunction. Each of these is connected to a specific organ in the body. In conditions of distress the Centre will start sending wrong information to the organ it controls, resulting in the formation of cancerous cells in the tissues.

Hamer found that when specific conflicts were resolved, the cancer immediately stopped growing at a cellular level. The dark spot dissolved and similar healing could also be seen around the, now inactive, cancerous tissue.

You experience a shock of fear: your hair stands on end, your heart starts pumping wildly and your muscles tense. A split-second after *that* your Emotional Brain has now started comparing what is known about the 'stick' with other emotional memories and 'reminds' you what worked best in those situations (e.g. run for your life!).

This is Bodymind intelligence at work and it is similar to a 'radar system' that tracks incoming aircraft, their size, their flight path and likely destination, automatically triggers a call to a flight centre, which in turn, ensures that a response is activated. The radar system is also programmed to ignore harmless phenomena such as clouds, birds and toy balloons, focusing purely on the immediate threat.

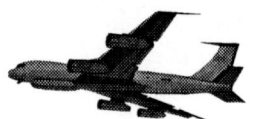

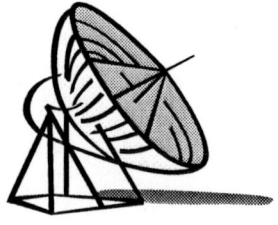

Bodymind radar rapidly scans the situations we are in and, just as rapidly, prepares an emotional or symptomatic response to let us know its views on what is going on.

Bodymind intelligence works on *information*. Information from the eyes and ears is picked up by the 'radar' system and cellular changes in the Emotional Brain, turn into chemical signals to the glandular system which, in turn, trigger physical changes in the rest of the body. In fact, Bodymind works just like a very sophisticated computer, except no computer has even been built that can mimic its flexibility, subtlety and power.

Just like a computer, the Emotional Brain also writes and stores away 'programs' for future use. Some of these programs recognise shapes, sounds and movements going on around you, while others match present experiences to other experiences that have happened to you in the past. The most important type of program, however, that concerns the production of symptoms is what we call a 'chemical memory'.

A chemical memory is stored away by Bodymind so that it can quickly recall what it has learnt about different experiences and how you responded to them. It then uses the memory to trigger the same set of emotions/symptoms you had before – every time that same situation comes up. Mostly, this is a useful, economical, mechanism that quickly reminds you what to do based on things you have learned to do in the past. It may keep you away from snakebite and save your life. It also keeps you motivated so that you persist with efforts that will bring you eventual satisfaction. So even though you don't *really* think you want to go to the gym tonight, a chemical memory released by the Emotional brain reminds you of the mild exhilaration and self-satisfaction that follows exercise, and off you go.

Some chemical memories automatically produce symptoms each time you come up against specific pressures. In the 'snake in the wood' example, given earlier, your Emotional Brain knew exactly what to do because it had prepared a chemical memory about strange-looking objects in the grass and was able to go into action in a split-second. The 'symptoms' of shock, although unpleasant, could have the effect of saving your life. The same goes for the other examples, given in Chapter 2, of your hairs standing on end while you are walking a dark street at night, or a mother's sudden arousal from sleep as her baby cries.

In other circumstances your Emotional Brain has 'learnt' that certain situations are unhealthy for you and, in its role as your guardian angel, seeks to protect you from harm.

Here are some other examples, this time taken from cases I have seen in Reverse therapy:

- *Karen* – symptoms of nausea, muscle ache and brain fog appeared whenever her partner came over from work and 'dumped' his worries, stress and fears on her. Emotionally, she found this extremely burdensome but felt unable to speak up for fear of offending her partner.

Candace Pert on the 'Molecules of Emotion'

Candace Pert has been writing and researching Mind-Body interactions for over twenty years. Her work on the chemistry of emotion reinforces the points made in this book about Bodymind intelligence and its use of 'chemical memories'.

She shows that once the Emotional brain has created an emotional response, the resulting state, along with information about the related situation, is stored not only by the Hippocampus but elsewhere in the body too, using what Dr Pert calls 'molecules of emotion'.

These are actually peptides (amino acid chains) that bind on to cells in the brain and, interestingly, over 95% of them can be found in the Hippocampus. These peptides travel all over the body but are especially strong in the spinal cord, the gut (the Enteric Nervous System), the skin, the muscles and in all the major glands. Not only does the Emotional brain 'tell' the glands, muscles and stomach what to do but they, in turn, feedback to it and let it know how they are 'feeling'. This information is then used by the Emotional Brain to either shut down the response, intensify it, or fine-tune it so that equilibrium can be maintained. No wonder Dr Pert writes:

> *'Mind doesn't dominate body, it becomes body – body and mind are one. I see in the process of [peptide] communication we have demonstrated, the flow of information through the whole organism, as evidence that the body is the actual outward manifestation, in physical space, of the mind'.*

- *Steve* – symptoms of fatigue, muscle ache and heart flutter came on whenever he went into his job as a school teacher only to come up against another day of over-work, in which he was already covering for a sick colleague (!) and had been given the job of marking all the exam papers for the form, as well as covering his own teaching schedule.

• *Eileen* – symptoms of acute pain in the neck, back and shoulders appeared during rows between her daughter, husband and grandson. She felt that she got no peace from the family rows, that no one considered her own need for peace and quiet, and felt powerless to intervene.

In each case, Bodymind had formed a chemical memory about the pressures coming on to the individual and each time those same pressures came up ('emotional dumping', 'overload of work from employer', 'family rows') the chemical memory was activated in order to produce warning symptoms and place the body on red alert. In the next chapter we will look at how Reverse Therapy solves this problem in detail. For now it is enough to note that Reverse Therapy aims at dissolving chemical memories by resolving the threats they are linked with.

The Hypothalamus – Bodymind's 'Master Controller'

Bodymind, as we have seen, is an incredibly clever thing. It does the complex job of protecting, motivating and guiding us, producing feelings, sensations, emotions and symptoms along the way, using a sophisticated information network that reaches every part of the body to do so. At the centre of this information network is the Hypothalamus, an organ the size of a small nut, which sits just underneath the Emotional Brain.[2]

The Hypothalamus controls every single part of your body through the glands. In particular, it regulates the Sympathetic Nervous System, which produces emotional changes, the Immune system, our defence against infection, and through the Adrenal glands, the action of the heart, muscles, skin and gut. It also directly controls your sleep function and internal temperature, physical growth and tissue renewal, and your appetite and sex drive.

---

[2] Some Neurologists question whether the Hypothalamus is in fact a gland because it doesn't actually produce any hormones. Instead it triggers the Pituitary gland to do this. However, because it controls every gland in the body it is convenient to think of it simply as a 'Master gland'.

45

The Hypothalamus is therefore the 'Master Controller' within your body. Like the captain of a ship it keeps everything running smoothly and reacts to any changes outside and inside the ship by altering its signals appropriately. The Hypothalamus, like our hypothetical captain, is also keenly receptive to the environment and ceaselessly receives information about it many times a second via inputs from the optic nerve, the Emotional Brain and the Thinking centres as well as from the rest of the body.

As a 'Master Controller' it works in a similar way to the thermostat on your central heating system: When your room gets too cold, the thermostat conveys that information to the furnace and turns it on. As your room warms up and the temperature gets beyond a certain set point, it sends a signal that tells the furnace to turn off. The Hypothalamus uses a variety of set-points to ensure that the organism is working at best possible capacity given the situation you are in. It has set-points for hunger, thirst, pain, pleasure, sexual satisfaction, anger/aggression and fear, as well as blood pressure, gut processes, Immune system responses, internal temperature, energy regulation and sleep. Unfortunately, these set-points can be thrown into chaos should the Hypothalamus become overwhelmed with messages from the Emotional brain, signalling that pressures are getting out of control, as is the case with the conditions known as Chronic Fatigue Syndrome/M.E. or Fibromyalgia.

The Hypothalamus also acts directly on the Sympathetic Nervous System through the Spinal cord to trigger the Alarm response that, in turn, creates a variety of physical changes that mobilise the body for action:

- Increase in heart rate.
- Dilation of the pupils.
- Stimulation of the sweat glands.
- Activation of muscle groups.
- Constriction of the blood vessels.
- Opening of bronchial tubes in the lungs.
- Inhibition of the digestive system

The other channel used by the Hypothalamus to control body function is through the glands. It signals the Pituitary to release hormones that, in turn, trigger hormone release in the Adrenal glands as well as in other glands such as the Thyroid, Thymus and Pancreas. The connection between the Hypothalamus-Pituitary-Adrenal glands is the most important in studying Chronic Fatigue Syndrome/M.E. and Fibromyalgia, because it is mainly through this pathway that the symptoms of these conditions are produced, as I will explain in Chapter 5. The pathway is known, for short, as the HPA axis.

Finally, the Hypothalamus stimulates the small nervous system in the gut. In fact, it is often in these nerves that you may first notice strong emotions. When you lose your appetite after hearing some bad news, get butterflies in your stomach before that first date, or you feel slightly sick after an argument, you are directly experiencing a communication from Bodymind through the HPA axis!

The Hypothalamus has three main functions:

1. It translates the emotional 'opinions' of the Emotional Brain into chemical messages that activate changes in the body.
2. It is continually fine-tuning the actions of the muscles, gut, heart, the Immune system, as well as many other functions, either firing them up or slowing them down, according to circumstances.
3. It tries to maintain 'homeostasis', meaning that it tries to keep the body in a state of balance. This is its most important function because it is only through the Hypothalamus that Bodymind can maintain a balance between environmental pressures and internal responses. Like the conductor of an orchestra, the Hypothalamus also harmonises the different body functions, smoothly switching resources from one area to another, ensuring that none of them hog the available energy and that all of them have what is needed to perform at maximum efficiency.

In healthy conditions the Hypothalamus sustains balance and ensures that we can swiftly adapt to changing circumstances. For example, energy is provided in the morning so that we can get going on the day's tasks but as night draws on, energy production dwindles as the Hypothalamus prepares us for rest and sleep. If we are in an emergency, digestion is stepped down as energy is switched to the muscles. If we catch a cold, Immune system production is prioritised but we may feel hot because the fight against infection is considered more important than maintaining a normal temperature.

In conditions of dis-ease the Hypothalamus is unable to carry out this balancing act, maintain its set-points or harmonise the work of the different functions in the body.

In general this happens when environmental pressures become overwhelming, creating urgent signals from the Emotional Brain to the Hypothalamus to do something about it. The Hypothalamus then sets in motion the General Adaptation Syndrome discovered by Hans Selye and which we discussed earlier but which we can now examine in more detail.

1. A series of demands, challenges, or burdens are picked up by the Emotional Brain and, through the Hypothalamus, emotions and low-level symptoms are created to warn the individual that they are at risk of harm.
2. Over time it becomes apparent that external pressures are increasing and no action has been taken. The Emotional Brain starts to track the situations and people linked to these pressures, signals the Hypothalamus to create the Alarm Reaction and creates a 'chemical memory' so that each time the same pressures come up the Alarm Reaction is triggered. This also acts to warn the individual that action to resolve the problem is required ever more urgently.
3. The Hypothalamus sees to it that the body works harder and harder in order to deal with the threat and send warning signals to the individual. More and more resources are being used up and the Hypothalamus is now struggling to maintain its balancing act.
4. By now, changes in the body-clock, over-work of the Sympathetic Nervous System, and destabilisation of the Immune system create non-specific symptoms such as fatigue, gut problems, headaches and recurrent infections. If

the individual still does not act and instead tries to fight the symptoms the Resistance stage gets under way.

5. During the Resistance stage the Hypothalamus, which constantly monitors the body through feedback, realises that the body is now struggling to cope. It interprets this as a fresh threat, presses the Alarm Reaction again to warn the individual, and works the body still harder. At the same time it changes the set-points in order to make economies. The sleep pattern is changed, energy decreases, metabolism slowed down and temperatures may fluctuate. Depending on the circumstances (the actual presence of infection, for example) The Immune system set-points may be raised or lowered.

6. The longer the situation goes on without corrective action, the more overactive the Hypothalamus becomes, in an increasingly desperate attempt to keep the body going in impossible conditions. The delicate feedback mechanisms between the Hypothalamus and the body functions break down as the body begins to 'give up' and the final, Stalemate stage, is reached..

At this point the Hypothalamus will continue to produce symptoms but must wait for further action from us in order to correct the imbalance. Once this has been done the Emotional Brain detects that the problem has been dealt with and can signal the Hypothalamus to return to normal function. And when *that* happens the symptoms can go. It is at this point that Reverse Therapy comes in.

Key points to remember:

- *Dis-ease is the state we get into when we lose our emotional balance under sustained pressure*
- *Hans Selye showed that dis-ease moves through 3 stages from uncomfortable emotions to minor, and then to major symptoms*
- *The Emotional Brain is the central control room of Bodymind*
- *When the 'radar system' in the Emotional Brain picks up that we are under threat for too long it triggers the Hypothalamus to trigger symptoms*
- *The Hypothalamus – the body's 'Master Controller' tries to keep a balance between external pressures and physical resources*
- *If this balance cannot be maintained the Hypothalamus re-creates the Alarm Reaction and sends symptoms to warn the individual action is required*

Chapter 4

What is Reverse Therapy?

In this chapter you will learn :

- ➤ Why Reverse Therapy is not a psychotherapy
- ➤ Main principles of Reverse Therapy
- ➤ That Reverse Therapy aims at dissolving chemical memories
- ➤ How Reverse Therapy dissolves symptoms

Reverse Therapy is not a psychotherapy

Reverse Therapy is a Bodymind healing process that reverses symptoms by working with them to understand their underlying Bodymind message. Although it has its roots in non-traditional forms of therapy it is not itself a psychotherapy. It does *not* assume that Chronic Fatigue Syndrome/M.E. or Fibromyalgia are psychological problems. They are glandular disorders that result from Bodymind's need to send symptoms to warn the individual that environmental pressures have not been dealt with and, using the Hypothalamus, to maintain the body on red alert until those pressures have been resolved. Reverse Therapy reverses these conditions by teaching clients to understand the link between situations that create pressure and what actions are required by Bodymind in order to resolve them.

When I came to give the name 'Reverse Therapy' to the approach, at the end of 2002, I wanted to include the word 'Reverse' in the title for three different reasons:

1. *Reversing attitudes to therapy.* Most forms of therapy assume that symptoms mean that there is something necessarily 'wrong' with the person. In fact many symptoms show that the opposite is true! Bodymind may have good reasons for producing symptoms and the fact

that it is communicating with us through them shows, at least, that it is working properly. By looking at why symptoms have become necessary we can help resolve them in a way that is more respectful of Bodymind.

2. *Reversing attitudes to symptoms* Instead of getting rid of them, Reverse Therapy sees symptoms as helpful allies. By paying attention to them, and the implied messages they contain, and then taking action on those same messages we can restore a state of healthy equilibrium in which symptoms are no longer necessary.

3. *Reversing symptoms.* Reverse Therapy is paradoxical. By *not* trying to control, or eliminate, or 'explain away' the symptoms – at least not directly – we find we get better results – we can work more quickly at resolving symptoms if we work with them instead of against them. This is because Bodymind responds much more quickly to a gentle, respectful approach that tries to understand its purposes than one that tries to ignore it.

The most important reason Reverse Therapy is not a psychotherapy is because we do not work with Headmind – its thoughts, dreams, memories and assumptions. Our focus is on Bodymind. Although we do not use massage or medication Reverse Therapists are concerned with the way that the body works, using its own intelligence. We educate our clients so that they understand why Bodymind uses chemical memories to produce symptoms and then we explain why Bodymind is forced to do this. We encourage them to become more aware of what is going on in their body and to become more finely attuned to their symptoms, and the situations in which they arise. We also encourage them to use awareness techniques, such as sensate focusing (see below) which enable them to develop Bodymind awareness.

Reverse Therapists also differ from the common view in psychotherapy that people have Unconscious Minds that store away unresolved emotions. It is Bodymind that does this. Working through an elaborate chain of hormones, cellular changes and peptide releases, Bodymind registers distressing experiences in the past and uses emotions and symptoms to let us know when it has been reactivated by situations occurring *in the present*. Such emotions and symptoms are not 'unconscious', although it is true that Headmind tries to ignore them or fight them. In many types of psychotherapy the focus is on *explaining* why people have problems in terms of 'unconscious' problems. In Reverse Therapy we consider that 'Headmind' explanations of this kind are practically useless and that the way to regain emotional health is to understand and act on Bodymind imperatives by acting in the *now*.

Principles of Reverse Therapy

Here are some of the most important principles behind our work. Understanding them will help make clearer to you how Reverse Therapy is effective in resolving the symptoms of Chronic Fatigue Syndrome/M.E. and Fibromyalgia.

Symptoms are a form of intelligent communication. Symptoms result from Bodymind activities that transfer information back and forwards between the Hypothalamus and the glands, the nervous system, the Immune system, the muscles, skin and gut. These are really changes in particular types of energy within the organism which we experience negatively only as long as we fail to understand that Bodymind is using this kind of communication as a last resort.

Attuning to Bodymind. We maintain a focus on Bodymind in every session and try to understand the important reasons Bodymind has for producing symptoms. We look at situations in which symptoms have been produced and ask ourselves the question: *'If I were this person's body what would I be trying to tell her/him about this situation?'* We continually direct the client to pay attention to their symptoms and get a feel for what Bodymind is asking them to do. Some clients may find this difficult to do at first because they are trying to fight symptoms by disconnecting from the pain/exhaustion that accompanies them. We seek to reverse this and help clients reconnect to Bodymind by staying with the symptoms until their function becomes clear.

Reverse Therapy is an educational process. We explain quite a lot about the Emotional Brain, the Hypothalamus and how symptoms get produced. By teaching them the facts about what is happening inside their bodies we dispel their fear of symptoms and make connections between specific situations and their Bodymind response. We thereby raise their awareness of Bodymind communication.

Symptoms are signs of 'dis-ease'. Symptoms are not necessarily evidence of 'illness'. In the initial stages at least they are signs that the individual is undergoing environmental pressures resulting in an imbalance between their personal needs and the demands placed on them. We encourage clients not to use terms like 'illness' or 'sickness' in describing their condition as this obscures the fact that Bodymind produces symptoms to protect and guide the individual.

Bodymind naturally promotes self-healing. Left to itself, without interference from unhealthy forms of Headmind or other people, Bodymind uses symptoms to deliver its felt opinion about problems, prepare us for action, and indicate what those actions should be. Its primary purpose is self-protection and the restoration of balance. It seeks to guide us towards the best possible state of adaptation to the environment. Once these purposes have been achieved it very naturally turns down the activities of the Hypothalamus and symptoms can then clear up.

Empathy and intuition. Reverse Therapists are trained to use the skills of empathy and intuition in order to understand the client's Bodymind. Empathy means putting oneself in someone else's place – in Reverse Therapy we identify with the client's body and develop a feel for what it is trying to express through emotions and symptoms. Intuition is closely related to empathy and refers to the ability to develop deep insights by noticing patterns in what people do. Intuition is usually 'unconscious' because we are not aware of how we developed the insight. In fact insight into another person's Bodymind comes about because our own Bodymind is subtly picking up clues from that person's facial expressions, voice tones, gestures, posture and the emphasis on particular words. Bodymind absorbs and processes all this information with astonishing speed, translating it into emotions until we are in a position to express the insight in words.

Reverse Therapy is evidence-based. The outcome of Reverse Therapy is that symptoms have been wholly or significantly resolved. Once the client has acknowledged, understood and acted on the symptom-message then Bodymind no longer has a need to maintain a chemical memory and produce symptoms. When the client acts on the symptom-message consistently the Emotional Brain picks up that environmental pressures are being successfully resolved and the Hypothalamus returns to its normal function of regulating and balancing body functions. The symptoms then disappear naturally and Reverse Therapy is concluded.

Using empathy and intuition in Reverse Therapy

Michael was twenty-two and had suffered from M.E. for six years. During the second session we were exploring the first appearance of his symptoms at the age of sixteen.

Michael recalled that his parents had gone through a bitter divorce when he was thirteen and, against his wishes, he had been forced to live with his Dad. Yet symptoms had not appeared until three years after that and there seemed to be no obvious connection to the symptoms.

Michael first noticed the symptoms while he was on a train journey to London, where he was due to reluctantly spend Xmas with relatives (he would rather have stayed in Manchester with his girlfriend). He was asked to recall sitting on the train as the symptoms came up.

He was struggling to understand what Bodymind was trying to 'tell' him on the train through the symptoms when I put myself 'in' his body at that time and sought to get a feel of what it was like to be on the train trying to communicate to Michael. Instantly, what came up for me was that the train journey was a re-run of the aftermath of the divorce, with Michael feeling forced to do something he did not want to do. I checked this insight with Michael and asked him to 'scan' his body with this communication in mind. Straight away he began to feel tearful and angry.

Following this discovery we were able to work on a Bodymind message that urged him to be more assertive with his family. With practice, his symptoms rapidly cleared.

Resolving symptoms

The 'symptoms' we are referring to here are the symptoms of reversible conditions linked to the state of dis-ease. Chronic Fatigue Syndrome, M.E. and Fibromyalgia are examples of such conditions. We are *not* referring to symptoms caused by infections, damage to tissue through injury or trauma, or triggered by genetic defect. Reverse Therapy is not suitable for such problems, which include conditions sometimes confused with Chronic Fatigue Syndrome, M.E and Fibromyalgia, such as Glandular Fever, Lyme Disease, Herpes viral complaints, Arthritis, Rheumatism, and Polymyositis.

Let us be clear that the symptoms of these conditions are not pleasant. Many of our clients experience them as painful, disabling and distressing. Nor do we underestimate the suffering this causes. Despite this, our first step in Reverse Therapy, after we have taught our clients how the symptoms are caused by the action of the Hypothalamus, is to teach them to look beyond the symptoms and to understand how Bodymind has no choice but to create them. This contrasts with most other approaches to Chronic Fatigue Syndrome/M.E. or Fibromyalgia, which try (and fail) to control or damp down symptoms.

Treatments which seek to remove or reduce symptoms of Chronic Fatigue Syndrome/M.E. or Fibromyalgia are misguided because they treat effects rather than causes. For example, Cortisone injections, which boost Cortisol levels and (supposedly) reduce Adrenal fatigue, are sometimes given to CFS patients, yet studies have shown that the benefits are marginal, at best, and that improvement may only be temporary. The reason this is so is that poor Adrenal function and low Cortisol levels are an effect, not the cause of the condition. So long as Bodymind continues to register that problematic situations have not been resolved then the Hypothalamus will continue to malfunction and so will the Adrenal glands. A similar problem relates to anti-depressants like Amitryptyline that are often prescribed for Fibromyalgia sufferers as well as for CFS in order to improve sleep, or to reduce pain. Again, long-term studies show that the benefits are very small, if they exist at all. This is borne out by my own findings in my conversations with clients, who tell me they notice no significant benefit. So long as the Hypothalamus is over-stimulated it will continue to produce a disturbed sleep cycle, and so long as the muscles continue to be over-worked by the HPA axis, then pain and muscle weakness will remain.

In Reverse Therapy, we call this attitude to symptoms 'shooting the messenger', meaning that, rather than deal with the real problem, we are simply taking out the bearer of bad news. It is rather like a car mechanic who, noticing that the thermometer on the dashboard keeps signalling that the car is over-heating, rips out the wires that work the thermometer instead of fixing the heating system.

Similar objections apply to the standard procedure known as 'pacing', which is offered in Cognitive-Behavioural therapy for M.E. Clients are instructed to ration their activities and take frequent rests in order to conserve energy. The objective is to reduce the fatigue symptoms. Again, the benefits are limited at best and are usually brief in duration. In some cases I have seen 'pacing' sometimes make the symptoms worse! This makes sense from a Reverse Therapy perspective for three reasons. The first is that avoiding activities may result in a Bodymind conclusion that the client is still more vulnerable than before, requiring still more symptoms to warn and protect the individual. The second is implied by the first: Bodymind requires *action* to resolve external problems. While 'resting' offers temporary relief from those problems, Bodymind remains aware that at some point the client must go back and encounter them again. The third reason is more subtle. The ultimate aim of Bodymind is to mobilise us towards a healthy, balanced, joyful involvement with life. A daily round in which people stay at home doing little and meeting no one, bored and perhaps depressed, living in fear of 'overdoing things' is likely to prompt fresh symptom communications from Bodymind.

Treatments that shoot down symptoms also make it much more difficult for clients (and their Reverse Therapists) to notice the symptoms as they come up and the situations they are linked with. Altogether, such treatments make it much harder to connect to Bodymind communications. This is one reason why, in Reverse

57

Therapy, we much prefer our clients not to take other treatments so long as they are working with us.

Reverse Therapy is unusual in that we are asking our clients to *reverse* their attitude to symptoms and take the first step in accepting that they are their for a purpose. Bodymind has no other way of adapting, protecting and warning them so long as problems are not resolved. One this first step is taken, clients can stop 'fighting' the symptoms and we can get on with the job of finding out what, specifically, Bodymind needs them to do.

Changing chemical memories

The key focus of Reverse Therapy is to dissolve the chemical memory that triggers symptoms. You may recall that chemical memories are stored in the Emotional Brain for three important reasons:

1. Bodymind uses this 'program' as an instant defence against external pressures.
2. Chemical memories put the body on red alert against the problem.
3. Bodymind uses this as a way of sending warning signals, in the form of symptoms, to the individual.

The more often situations linked to the chemical memory come up, the stronger that chemical memory becomes. As this happens the symptoms may also become stronger or more deeply embedded. Conversely, when actions are taken to deal with those pressures the less need Bodymind has for that chemical memory. It is less and less activated until it weakens and fades away. When it dissolves completely then the symptoms will dissolve with it.

To a lesser degree, Bodymind creates numerous chemical memories linked to different emotional states right throughout our lives. Some of these may still be with you now while others are faded away and long-forgotten. For example, babies form a chemical memory of threat if they are hungry and go too long without feeding. This provokes them to cry and yell with frustration. Yet I doubt whether

58

there are many readers of this book who throw a tantrum if their dinner is delayed! This is because, over time, most of you learned to appreciate that, eventually, your milk would come! The 'threat' disappeared and the automatic symptom of rage disappeared with it.

Similarly, you may have been nervous about learning to drive a car. A chemical memory formed which triggered a fit of nerves each time you took the wheel. This was really Bodymind warning you to take it easy and drive slowly until your confidence reached the right level. It may also have been telling you to make sure you had the right instructor! Gradually, and beyond the milestone of passing your driving test, you learned to drive a car safely and, again, the threat was resolved. Now, each time you took the wheel there may have been a mild feeling of satisfaction. This state replaced the old chemical memory until Bodymind had no further use for it (unless you had a crash before this could happen – in which case Bodymind kept the chemical memory for a while longer until confidence was restored).

Small-scale pressures need not lead to lasting symptoms. Pressures by themselves do not cause illness because our bodies are remarkably resilient. Bodymind, and its mechanisms for adaptation, coping and survival, sees to that. It is when pressures are allowed to stack up and go ignored that we develop a problem. This usually happens either when we are overwhelmed by life-events, or when we suffer from Headmind blocks that lead to the sense that we do not have permission to act as we should for the sake of our own health. In fact, dis-ease – the state we get into when pressures continue and, because we have lost our connection with Bodymind – is really a state in which we have lost our basic sense of who we are and what we could be. Reverse Therapy addresses this by encouraging clients to attune to their deepest emotional needs and discover opportunities of fulfilling them.

A chemical memory is most often linked to an emotionally painful event that contains basic Bodymind learning about self, life or others. It is also linked to an overwhelming need or desire. For example, another client, whom I shall call 'Sian' reported early-warning symptoms of recurrent fatigue and brain fog when she moved to a new home in a remote part of Scotland. Her husband's job had taken him there and she agreed that 'it was for the best'. Yet Sian loved the home she had before, where all her friends were, where her daughter was too, and where she was happy. Soon, she found herself without friends and with nothing to do except take walks on her own in the countryside. Sian was soon very bored and lonely, and her symptoms steadily became worse. Interestingly, she recalled being in a similar position as a child when her parents had moved from England to Scotland – she had hated that move and had wept for months at the loss of all her friends from school. Somewhere along the way, it seemed, Bodymind had preserved a chemical memory of that loss, and her sense of powerlessness at the time. That memory had become reactivated at the move, this time more seriously resulting in symptoms. Sian eventually became well, but only after taking up the courage to talk to her husband about her need to spend more time with her friends and with her daughter.

Diagram of chemical memory in dis-ease

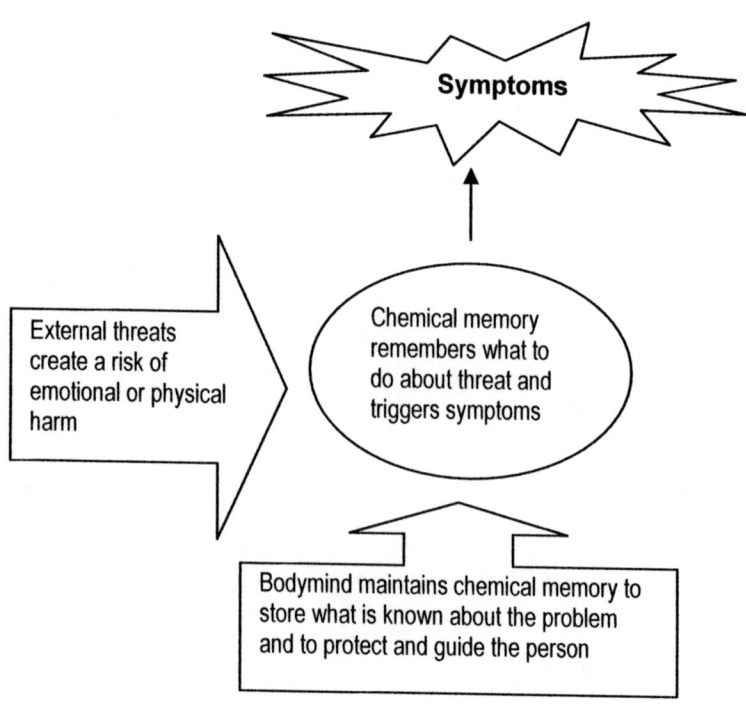

Examples of challenging life-events which may lead Bodymind to form a chemical memory include:

- Abuse, alcoholism and violence.
- Rejection and loss.
- The strain of supporting other people.
- Conflict and bullying.
- Excessive work-loads.
- Marital struggles.
- Hassles from family members.
- Unresolved fear arising from accidents, assault and shock.
- Pressure arising from changes in education and career.
- Financial disasters.
- Deprivation – poverty, low opportunities, and isolation.

Once again it is important to stress that timely action can abolish Bodymind's need to maintain a chemical memory and send symptoms. We saw with Sian that the solution was for her to deal with the pressure of changing homes was for her to maintain contact with her friends and family. But to do that she needed to re-learn how to speak up about her needs with her husband.

No one person's problems are ever alike and for that reason Bodymind requires different things from each individual. But common solutions include:

- Being more open with other people
- Making more personal time for oneself
- Becoming more assertive about one's needs
- Getting support from other people
- Developing new personal skills
- Saying 'No' more often
- Setting limits to involvement in draining situations
- Spending more time on fulfilling activities
- Reconsidering work commitments
- Restoring confidence in difficult situations

Diagram of recovery in Reverse therapy

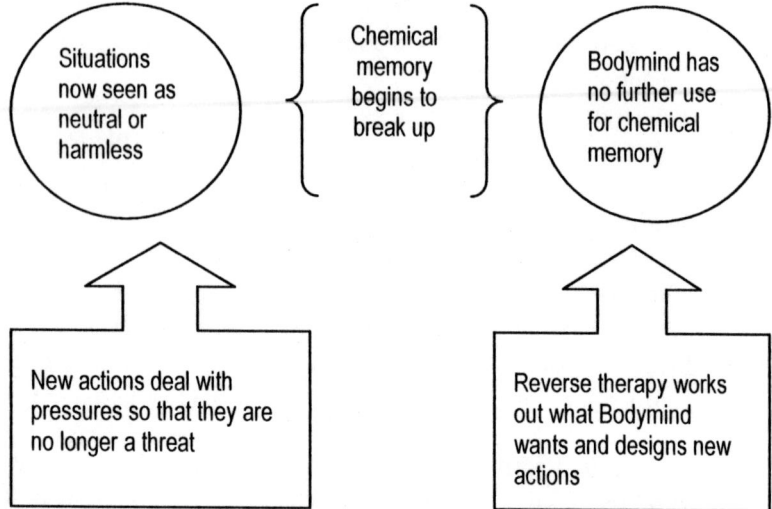

Reverse therapy helps clients recover health by first identifying the pressures linked to the chemical memory, working out what it is Bodymind wants done, and then designing the new actions to take. Throughout, we act as a source of support and encouragement, while keeping the focus firmly on Bodymind communication.

Key points to remember:

➢ Reverse Therapy is not a psychotherapy because it works with Bodymind, not Headmind
➢ Reverse Therapy abolishes symptoms by dissolving the chemical memories that trigger them
➢ Chemical memories are created by Bodymind to preserve important information about external pressures, and what needs to be done about them
➢ When clients understand and act on what Bodymind is trying to tell them through the symptoms, the chemical memory dissolves and the symptoms disappear with them

Chapter 5

About Chronic Fatigue Syndrome,/M.E. and Fibromyalgia

In this chapter you will learn:

> - That CFS/M.E. and Fibromyalgia have been around for a long time
> - That they are non-specific illnesses that can only be diagnosed indirectly
> - That there may be over 1 million cases in the United Kingdom
> - That the direct physical cause of these conditions is overwork of the Hypothalamus, or 'Hypothalamitis'

These conditions are not new.

In 1869 a condition was identified by George Beard, an American neurologist, which he called 'Neurasthenia'. The symptoms originally classified for this illness were physical exhaustion, headaches, muscle tremors, extreme sensitivity to noise and light, sleep disturbance, and poor concentration.

Beard considered it that it was caused by too many demands on the Nervous system. He pointed out that regimented work, commuting, unstable employment and the increasing speed of life were creating ever too many pressures on people. He argued that these pressures, if left unattended, gradually depleted the reserves of 'nervous energy' in people, leading to illness. A Neurasthenic, he said, was a person who had used up these reserves and had gone into 'nervous bankruptcy'. He prophesied that, as the industrialisation of the world proceeded, such cases would become more and more frequent. Indeed, there was an explosion of diagnosed cases throughout Europe in the last thirty years of the nineteenth century.

Although Neurasthenia was generally recognised, there were no adequate explanations for why the symptoms appeared and nor was there a cure. The usual 'treatment' was seclusion and rest which, then as now, can only provide temporary relief for the symptoms.

As a result of this lack of understanding, 'Neurasthenia' was too often mixed up with other conditions and, as a result, the term quickly became over-used and was eventually dropped as it became too vague a label to be useful. Also, Sigmund Freud, who treated several cases, regarded the condition as 'psychological' and because there were no tests for Neurasthenia that could lead to a diagnosis of a physical complaint, his view was generally accepted. Thereafter many sufferers were often dismissed as 'hysterical'. This dismissal, using different terms, continues to this day with most unfortunate effects.

Florence Nightingale

A famous case of Neurasthenia was that of Florence Nightingale, the founder of the nursing profession in the UK. She made her reputation during the Crimean War (1854-56) in which she went out to nurse the British war casualties in traumatic conditions. The death rate from injuries was 40%, a figure Florence, by means of superhuman efforts based on sanitation, reorganization of the hospitals, and intensive personal care of the soldiers, brought down to 2%. In 1856 she came home but from then on was always ill with what was then a poorly understood condition. Her symptoms were fatigue, muscle weakness, headaches, nausea, breathlessness and heart palpitations – all now consistent with a diagnosis of Chronic Fatigue Syndrome. Despite her illness Florence continued to over-work, this time campaigning to get the government to built properly-built hospitals and staff them with trained nurses. She steadily became worse and was eventually bed-ridden for 6 years. Although she made some improvement she never fully recovered.

Given that human beings have not changed much, in biological terms, for many millennia, it is likely that the conditions now known as Chronic Fatigue Syndrome/M.E. and Fibromyalgia have been around for a long time but have not been recognised as such. They would arise whenever human beings were exposed to intolerable pressures, in societies which did not promote Bodymind health. The fact that this has been the case in the West for over a hundred years now probably explains the rapidly escalating number of reported cases.

Unfortunately, the labels now used to describe the illness are no more helpful than the 'Neurasthenia' diagnosis was. None of them explain how the illness is caused and nor do they point to the cure.

Let us look at some of these labels:

- Fibromyalgia – a name that means 'pain in the muscles and connective tissues of the joints' – which is merely a description of one of the main symptoms.

- Chronic Fatigue Syndrome – again this is just a description of one of the symptoms.

In neither case does the diagnostic label reveal any information about the cause of the disorder. This gives rise to a lot of frustration, as my clients frequently tell me, as they often leave the doctor's surgery or the hospital with little more than the label. It is rather like someone going to a medical doctor to get treatment for a persistent sore throat and being told that they have 'Sore Throat Syndrome' and that there is no cure!

- Myalgic Encephalomyelitis (M.E.). This label does try to state the cause but unfortunately it happens to be wrong. The term means 'painful inflammation of the brain and spinal cord'. We now know that no such inflammation exists and use of the label has now been discouraged in the UK (although it is still widely used.)

Diagnosing these conditions

Chronic Fatigue Syndrome/M.E.

The major problem in diagnosing these illnesses is that no reliable physical tests exist which can accurately identify it. This is why they are referred to as 'non-specific' illnesses (which means that no-one has yet worked out how to diagnose them properly!).

Identification of the problem relies heavily ruling out other illnesses first. This is known as a 'diagnosis of exclusion' and is based on simple blood and urine tests, and also, in some cases, on laboratory tests. These rule out conditions such as Thyroid problems, Kidney/Liver dysfunction, Anaemia, Diabetes and Arthritis, any of which can cause similar symptoms to those of the disorder. Once that has been done a diagnosis based on the symptoms themselves can go ahead.

In the case of CFS/M.E., the first step is to clinically evaluate the presence of chronic fatigue, i.e. self-reported persistent or relapsing fatigue lasting six or more consecutive months, which is not substantially alleviated by rest, and which results in substantial reduction in previous levels of occupational, educational, social or personal activities.

Additionally, a diagnosis is achieved on the basis of four or more of the following symptoms, all of which must have persisted or recurred during six or more consecutive months of illness and must not have predated the fatigue:

- Sore throat
- Swollen glands
- Muscle pain
- Joint pain without joint swelling or redness
- Headaches of a new type
- Unrefreshing sleep
- Post-exertional malaise lasting more than twenty-four hours.
- Nausea
- Gut problems
- Light/noise sensitivity
- Dizziness
- Fluctuating temperatures
- Impairment in short term memory or concentration

According to David Jameson, in his book, *Mind-Body Health and Stress Tolerance*, there are about 6 symptoms that are experienced by most patients:

- Fatigue: 95-100%
- Nausea: 60-90%
- Irritable Bowel Syndrome: 50-90%
- Low blood pressure: 86%
- Sleep disorders: 65-100%
- Sensitivity to light: 65-90%

Prevalence

One of the earliest attempts to estimate the prevalence of CFS was conducted by the Centers for Disease Control and Prevention in the USA from 1989 to 1993. The study estimated that between 4.0 and 8.7 per 100,000 persons eighteen years of age or older have CFS and are under medical care. However it is likely these were underestimates due to the fact that many sufferers do not report their symptoms to their medical doctors.

A more recent study in Seattle estimated that CFS affects between 75 and 265 people per 100,000 of the population, while another study from San Francisco put the occurrence of 'CFS-like disease' (i.e. both reported/diagnosed and unreported cases) at approximately 200 per 100,000 persons. If this is so then there would exist about 1.2 million cases in the UK and over 4 million cases in the USA

The condition occurs in all ethnic groups and social classes to the same extent, affects almost twice as many women as men, with the commonest age of onset between the early twenties and mid-forties. According to the report, children as young as five can develop the condition. The commonest age of onset for this group is between thirteen and fifteen years although, overall, most sufferers are between the ages of twenty and forty.

Fibromyalgia Syndrome (FMS)

Along with many other researchers, we consider that FMS and Chronic Fatigue Syndrome/M.E. are expressions of the same disorder. In fact the symptoms listed above for CFS/M.E, are the same as for Fibromyalgia. The main difference is that, where fatigue is often mentioned as the dominant symptoms for CFS/M.E., muscle/joint pain is listed as the main symptom in FMS. On the basis of my clinical observations I hypothesise, also, that many patients with an FMS label tend not to have Immune system disorders, where CFS/M.E patients are more likely to report sore throat, swollen glands and feverishness – all linked to

---

CFS/M.E. and Fibromyalgia are not Depression!

There is a view held by some that these problems are really forms of Clinical Depression. This view is both insulting as well as wrong. In fact the symptoms of Depression are very different – the most important one being that, while Cortisol levels are often high in Depression, they are low in these problems.

The reason many people with these conditions are in fact depressed is due to their experience of illness – including the fact that they may have been told their problems are all in the mind!

The experience of having a disabling illness for which people have been told there is no cure is profoundly dispiriting and will give rise to a variety of painful emotions. As we shall see, these emotions are often 'de-pressed' purely in order that the sufferer can 'keep going' in impossible conditions. Unfortunately, the result is that *all* emotions are depressed, including the hopeful ones. This simply adds to the underlying problem of despair.

Reverse Therapy addresses both the illness and any accompanying Depression.

Immune system problems. However, that may be, both conditions have the same root in over-work of the HPA axis which impacts on the Immune system and the Muscular-skeletal system in different ways.

According to the National Institute of Health in the USA, Fibromyalgia affects about 3.7 million Americans, which would indicate an incidence of 170 per 100,000 of the population. If this is so, that would mean there are about 975,000 sufferers in the United Kingdom.

Post-Viral Fatigue Syndrome (PVFS)
Again, this is yet another term for the same condition as CFS/M.E. and FMS. It is used as a separate label by some specialists who labour under the mistaken view that the condition is caused by a viral infection, the main culprit usually being the Epstein-Barr virus, which causes Glandular Fever. This despite the fact that no virus has ever been identified as common to all patients.

As we shall see later in this chapter these viral infections are an effect, not a cause, of the disorder. As the HPA axis progressively over-works, Immune system breakdown often occurs, leading to the entry of opportunistic viruses. The fact that this problem typically occurs early on in the condition has led to this confusion between effects and causes. But the fact that a viral infection is one of the first symptoms does not mean that it is a cause! If that kind of thinking were true then having a high temperature would be the cause of the common cold!

What causes Chronic Fatigue Syndrome/M.E./Fibromyalgia?

In this chapter I argue that Chronic Fatigue Syndrome/M.E., Fibromyalgia and PVFS are all expressions of the same disorder and that the source of the problem lies in the wrong work of the Hypothalamus. Behind that, Bodymind intelligence is seeking to warn, protect and mobilise the individual against threat, using the Hypothalamus for this purpose. The symptoms are created partly by the Alarm Reaction, partly by Bodymind's use of symptoms as warning signals, and partly from a breakdown in feedback between the Hypothalamus and the Adrenal glands.

Because over-work of the Hypothalamus is the root, physical cause of the symptoms, Reverse therapists give the convenient name 'Hypothalamitis' to the problem. This, at least, has the merit of indicating the cause of the condition and also hints at the cure – once Bodymind is satisfied that environmental pressures have been dealt with, it can quickly signal for the Hypothalamus to go back to normal function.

At this point I need to make it clear that 'Hypothalamitis' is a serious physical illness created in the Central Nervous System and is most certainly not a psychological problem. Its symptoms are created automatically by reflex neurochemical reactions that lead to disorders in the HPA axis. Our clients are certainly not conscious of these complex neurochemical changes and (unless they enter Reverse Therapy) are unable to control them.

The essential steps in the illness are as follows:

1. Environmental pressures are experienced by the individual.
2. Pressures escalate and low-level emotions and symptoms are not picked up and acted upon, leaving the pressures unresolved.
3. The Emotional Brain signals the Hypothalamus to create an Alarm Reaction, thus increasing and intensifying symptoms.
4. If pressures are still not resolved a 'chemical memory' associated with those pressures is created by the Emotional Brain.
5. Each time the same pressures come along, the chemical memory triggers a fast release of messages to the Hypothalamus.
6. Over time the Hypothalamus works harder and harder to put the body on 'red alert' and to signal through the symptoms that corrective action is required.
7. If no corrective action is taken, the HPA axis continues to be stimulated and the Immune system, the Sympathetic Nervous System, the muscles and gut become seriously over-worked.
8. Eventually the Adrenal glands and Immune system become destabilised and cease to respond to the ever-increasing demands from the Hypothalamus (Resistance phase)
9. The Hypothalamus is unable to perform its subtle balancing act and ceases to regulate major body functions effectively. Feedback mechanisms break down and the symptoms become chronic (Stalemate phase)

The cause of the condition lies originally in the Emotional Brain, linking through the Hypothalamus and then on to the HPA axis, which, in turn, creates each of the symptoms.

Flowchart showing development of 'Hypothalamitis'

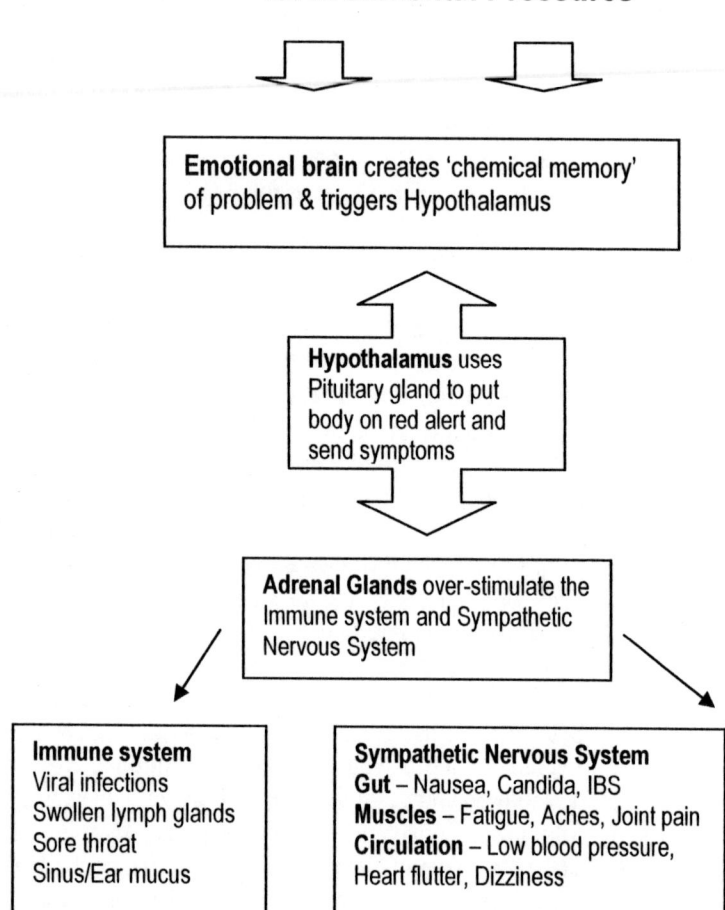

Environmental Pressures

Emotional brain creates 'chemical memory' of problem & triggers Hypothalamus

Hypothalamus uses Pituitary gland to put body on red alert and send symptoms

Adrenal Glands over-stimulate the Immune system and Sympathetic Nervous System

Immune system
Viral infections
Swollen lymph glands
Sore throat
Sinus/Ear mucus

Sympathetic Nervous System
Gut – Nausea, Candida, IBS
Muscles – Fatigue, Aches, Joint pain
Circulation – Low blood pressure, Heart flutter, Dizziness

Step-by-step guide to 'Hypothalamitis' symptoms

CFS/M.E./FMS are complex conditions and this account is necessarily simplified. The intention here is to help readers with these conditions understand how and why they occur. It is hoped that this explanation will help dispel the mystery surrounding these conditions. That done, much of the fear connected to the symptoms can be swept away.

Reference can be made to the flowchart on the previous page to aid understanding.

Muscle weakness/Pain
This symptom is caused by over-stimulation of the muscles due to the release of Adrenal hormones. As the muscles work harder and harder (even while the person is at 'rest') this leads to a build up of lactic acid, which quickly disperses, causing the characteristic aching reported by so many sufferers. Continuous muscle tension also creates post-exertional malaise as the exhausted muscles take longer to recover from the extra work they are asked to perform.

In normal conditions the Hypothalamus would detect that the muscles were exhausted and would turn down the 'thermostat'. But when 'Hypothalamitis' takes over it perceives the increase in fatigue as a sign that the muscles are struggling to cope. It therefore increases the demand on the Adrenal glands to make them work harder in order to avoid another emergency. The result is a vicious spiral in which exhaustion prompts ever-increasing demands for more effort, leading to yet more exhaustion…

Headaches
See above. This is a special case of one muscle – the scalp muscle – overworking and creating pressure on the skull.

Joint pain
Research has not shown that there is any clear-cut malfunction in the joints in CFS/M.E./FMS cases. It is therefore more likely that the true problem lies in over-exertion of the muscles, leading to referred pain in the fibrous tissue that connects the muscles to the bone around the joints.

Chronic Fatigue
Again, this is linked to over-exertion of the muscles. Research shows also that the Mitochondria in the muscle fibres – which act as 'furnaces' that convert glucose into energy – cease to work properly under the strain of constant demands from the Hypothalamus. This naturally adds to the general feeling of exhaustion.

Decreased concentration/short term memory ('Brain fog')
This is likely to have several causes. One is the general exhaustion that follows muscle fatigue. Another is a malfunction of the Hippocampus, in the Emotional brain which processes short-term memories. When sleep is disturbed the Hippocampus is unable to clear the memories, leading to overload and then to shut-down.

Sleep disturbance
The Hypothalamus contains an area that controls our 'body clock' and regulates the sleep cycle. In normal circadian activity (i.e. changes from activity to rest over a 24-hour period) the Hypothalamus ensures that we achieve an adequate balance between rest and activity. In the condition known as 'Hypothalamitis' this balance is disturbed leading either to Hypersomnia (too much sleep) or Insomnia (too little).

My clinical observation is that reduced sleep function is far more common than Hypersomnia. The two figures below explain this.

In healthy conditions the circadian rhythm generated in the brain should look like this:

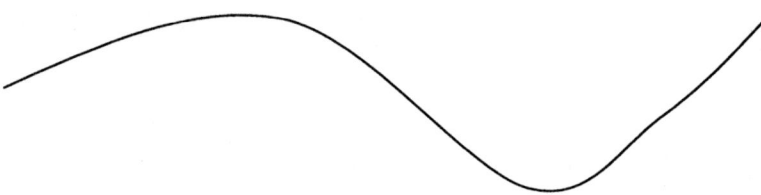

This is a 'slow' wave that contains deeper troughs making it easier for the person to remain asleep. As Hypothalamitis sets in and disturbs sleep function, however, the wave looks more like this:

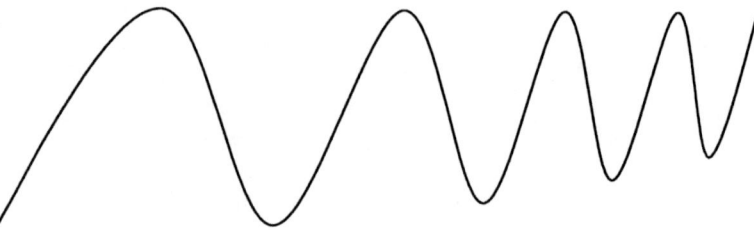

Each 'bottom' is much narrower, leaving little time for the

individual to settle in to or remain in sleep.

Fluctuating temperatures
This has a similar cause to sleep disturbance as temperature is controlled directly by the Hypothalamus. Inside the Hypothalamus are thermo-receptor cells which act like the thermostat on a central heating system – when the cells register a fall/rise in blood temperature they trigger a release of hormones to increase/decrease the burn-up of glucose, change the action of the sweat glands and open or close the skin pores. If the feedback mechanism in the HPA axis breaks down the Hypothalamus ceases to do its proper job of adjusting internal feelings of heat and cold.

Viral/bacterial infections
Many people with 'Hypothalamitis' succumb to viral infections at the start of their illness. This viral problem is *not* the cause of 'Hypothalamitis' but one of its effects. In the initial stages of the condition the Immune system works very hard at producing antibodies to defend against infections. After a time, unable to keep up this kind of response, the Immune system breaks down and opportunistic viruses then either enter the system or are activated inside the body. An example of the latter type is Epstein-Barr virus that causes Glandular Fever. In fact most of us carry this virus; it just never gets activated. In 'Hypothalamitis' the virus may be activated following breakdown in the Immune system, leading to the mistaken view that this virus goes on to cause CFS/M.E.

Flu-like aches/Feverishness
This is also linked to over-activity of the Immune system. A common report I hear from my clients is that they feel as if they were always just about to 'come down' with an illness that never actually materialises, rather like the feeling one has in the first few hours of a cold/flu infection. The aching/feverishness is caused by increased levels of antibodies resulting from an Immune system on constant 'red alert'.

Swollen lymph glands/sore throat
These symptoms are often – mistakenly – offered as evidence that CFS/M.E. are post-viral conditions as they are linked to the actions of the Immune system when it fights infection. In 'Hypothalamitis'

the Immune system is prompted to remain on 'action stations' against infection – even where no threat exists. The Immune system periodically increases production of lymphatic fluid, thereby swelling the lymph glands. Antibodies are diverted to the throat and create inflammation.

Dizziness

This is created by a combination of factors. Activation of the Sympathetic Nervous System causes reduced blood pressure which is particularly noticeable when the individual stands up too quickly. Reduced blood sugar (caused by diversion of glucose to the muscles) also creates a light-headed feeling that adds to the problem. In some cases the Immune system can create excess mucus in the sinuses, leading to a build-up of fluid in the middle ear – which regulates our sense of balance. Finally, 'Hypothalamitis' can lead to reduced vasoconstriction of the blood vessels supplying the heart and the limbs. Over a prolonged period of time, this effect may cause gravitational pooling in the leg veins, which increases orthostatic intolerance.

Gut problems/Irritable bowel

The gut is stimulated through the Sympathetic Nervous System. In 'Hypothalamitis', the gut responds by going on 'red alert' and stepping up its reactivity to toxins in the diet – even where no toxins exist, or where they would otherwise be easily tolerated. This leads to an increase in stomach acid, increased bowel contractions, and inflammation of the bowel wall.

Nausea

See above. This is most probably linked to increased production of stomach acid.

Candida Albicans

Increased sensitivity to food compounds leads to an imbalance of acid/alkali in the intestine leading to decreased control over the naturally occurring flora in the gut, known as Candida. Also, the Immune system, when working properly, controls the growth of Candida but, in 'Hypothalamitis', is unable to do so.

This problem is wrongly held by some to be 'the cause' of

CFS/M.E. and antibiotics may be prescribed that do more harm than good. These further impair the already disturbed control functions exercised by the gut and Immune system, and the Candida symptoms return worse than before.

'Hypothalamitis' and the Immune system

'Hypothalamitis' sufferers have both over-active and under-active Immune system responses, which work in different ways. Both relate to a breakdown in control over the Immune system.

The Immune system is actually a complex of interlocking processes in which the HPA axis, the cells, Cytokines (messengers that tell the cells which antibodies to produce) and the antibodies that destroy invaders all play a part in the defence against infection.

The body defends itself against infections in two different ways known as the Th1 and Th2 responses. If the body is threatened by viruses and bacteria coming from the outside then Natural Killer (NK) cells are created to eliminate them (the Th1 response). If the problem occurs inside the body (cancers, infected host cells, fungi, etc.) then T-cells are created to identify and destroy them (Th2 response). In normal conditions the body can switch from one mode of attack to the other and quickly return the Immune system to rest, waiting on standby until the next threat emerges.

As 'Hypothalamitis' develops, however, the Adrenal glands overwork and eventually cease to respond to the Hypothalamus. Cortisol is the main hormone produced by the Adrenals to manage the Immune system and return it to balance. As less and less Cortisol is produced, the balance is lost and the individual either develops either an exaggerated Th1 response or Th2 response.

If the sufferer is Th1-active then the Immune system will overwork to fight colds, flu and other viruses. But its ability to control chemical sensitivities, allergies (including food intolerance) and yeasts (such as Candida) will weaken. In Th-2 over-activity the reverse is the case.

How fear of illness worsens the symptoms

'Hypothalamitis' begins when Bodymind, working through the Emotional Brain, considers that the individual is overwhelmed by environmental pressures and that no solution appears to be in sight. If the condition is prolonged, however, a further problem emerges – the experience of feeling ill, disabled and distressed creates yet more environmental pressure!

Let us also mention the common experiences of many sufferers from CFS/M.E./FMS in which they are dismissed as 'hypochondriacs', or told their symptoms are 'all in the mind'. They may be informed by other consultants that they have an incurable viral or neural condition for which there is no remedy. They trudge wearily from one consulting room to the next, trying one 'cure' after another but with no success. And each failure breeds fresh hopelessness and fear. This is in fact the reason why so many sufferers get depressed – only to be told by some consultants that their condition is in fact a form of Depression! They are then prescribed Anti-depressants which do little to alleviate the symptoms, leading to fresh disappointment and a renewed fear that they will never get well. At the same time they are likely to be suffering from financial problems as they give up work which, in turn leads to increased stress in the home as their families struggle to get by on a reduced income. Activities which gave them joy, fulfilment and a sense of purpose are given up as they feel too exhausted to continue with them, increasing the negative emotions they have about their condition.

They may suffer from incomprehension, ridicule and rejection from employers, friends and family members, which deepens their despair and loneliness. At this point they may try to fight or ignore the symptoms in an effort to be seen as 'normal' again, only to find that with each effort their symptoms worsen. Lastly, the sufferer's situation is worsened by the fact that symptoms come and go, with 'good' days unpredictably followed by 'bad' days; some symptoms disappearing (perhaps returning months later) only to be replaced by new symptoms.

The fresh pressures created by the experience of illness,

hopelessness and rejection then create further changes in the Emotional Brain and HPA axis which intensify the symptoms. Here is an explanation for how this happens:

Because sufferers so desperately want to get well and be free of symptoms they become very sensitive to the appearance of symptoms, frequently checking their bodies to establish whether symptoms have returned or got worse. After a while this 'checking' response becomes a habit and is picked up by the Emotional Brain as a sign that fear and pressure have returned. When the Emotional Brain notices that we have become anxious about the symptoms and are 'checking' again it concludes that we are vulnerable and triggers a fresh Alarm Reaction to the Hypothalamus. Eventually, another chemical memory is created – this time for the experience of illness!

'Hypothalamitis' is now triggered by two chemical memories – the environmental pressures that created the condition in the first place plus the symptoms themselves! This weird loop creates a trap in which every time 'Hypothalamitis' symptoms are produced the resulting state of fear produces still more symptoms. In an attempt to cope with illness the individual often shuts himself off from the outside world out of fear – which then prompts the Emotional Brain to activate the 'Hypothalamitis' state all over again. What is worse, each time the response occurs it intensifies each chemical memory and makes them more likely to activate.

This trap is known as a 'negative feedback loop' and is possibly the reason that some sufferers experience the same level of symptoms day after day in a wearying round of pain, discomfort and exhaustion. It is also the reason why so many people find recovery difficult. In the next chapter we will look at how Reverse Therapy resolves this negative loop.

Key points to remember:

> ➤ Chronic Fatigue Syndrome/M.E. and Fibromyalgia illnesses are probably as old as the human race
> ➤ CFS/M.E. and FMS are all different forms of the same condition – 'Hypothalamitis'
> ➤ The cause of these conditions is chronic overwork of the Hypothalamus
> ➤ Each and every symptom can be explained and traced back through the HPA axis to the Hypothalamus
> ➤ 'Hypothalamitis' continues so long as the Emotional Brain needs to maintain a chemical memory to put the body on red alert and send warning symptoms
> ➤ Fear of the symptoms leads the Emotional Brain to create another chemical memory that produces still more symptoms to warn the individual not to be afraid of the symptoms and to work with them

Chapter 6

Reverse Therapy for M.E./Chronic Fatigue Syndrome and Fibromyalgia

In this chapter you will learn:

> ➤ The importance of correct diagnosis
> ➤ What case histories show about chemical memories
> ➤ How we help clients understand Bodymind
> ➤ About deciphering symptom-messages
> ➤ The way to overcome fear and depression
> ➤ How clients return to normal life
> ➤ How to prepare for the first session

The first steps

The first steps towards the cure are carried out during the first two sessions. These form an introduction to Reverse Therapy and also enable the therapist to gain an understanding of how the client's Bodymind works and what it is trying to teach the client through the symptoms.

Checking the diagnosis. Because CFS/M.E. and Fibromyalgia are non-specific conditions (which means that no-one has yet worked out how to diagnose them properly!) it is important that the Reverse Therapist checks for a diagnosis of exclusion. This is based on simple blood and urine tests, and also laboratory tests. These rule out other conditions such as Thyroid problems, Kidney/Liver dysfunction, Anaemia, Diabetes and Arthritis, any of which can cause similar symptoms to those of the disorder. This exclusion of other problems enables Reverse Therapy to go ahead on the assumption that our client's condition is the result of 'Hypothalamitis'.

Case history. The Reverse Therapist takes a careful case history of the illness, tracing back to the very first appearance of the symptoms. Often this is not the same moment in time as the client first became aware of feeling ill. This is because symptoms develop gradually at first and may not have been noticed at the start for what they were. For example, many clients tell us that they experienced fatigue spells for months, or even years, before they went for diagnosis. Nor do many of our clients realise that they were in fact suffering from 'Hypothalamitis' until we point it out to them. Another example of an early symptom that may not be recognised as part of the condition is Immune system weakness, leading to a series of infections and viral problems.

It is vital that we identify, as closely as possible, the real start of the problem because then we can look at the environmental pressures that were going on then and work out what it was that Bodymind was reacting to. For that reason, once we have taken a list of symptoms, we often ask questions like:

> *'And did you notice any of these symptoms there, way before you really became aware of feeling ill?'*

> *'Were any of these symptoms there in a very faint form earlier than that?'*

> *'What was the very first beginning of the beginning of these symptoms?'*

Consideration of the case history then passes to a review of the life-events that were present just before, and during, first symptom appearances. What the Reverse Therapist keeps continually in mind while this investigation continues are two inter-related factors:

> 1. 'What pressures was the client coming up against and what would have been needed to resolve them?'

> 2. 'How was Bodymind trying to adapt the client to these pressures and what was it trying to communicate through the symptoms?'

Explaining 'Hypothalamitis'. We explain to our clients how their symptoms are produced through the action of the Hypothalamus working through the HPA axis, using one of our diagrams for this purpose.

This is important because it is usually the first time our clients have met with a comprehensive explanation for their illness. Indeed, many of them tell us that just listening to this explanation creates an enormous relief, followed by a rapidly dawning realisation of the cure. We tell them that understanding how the symptoms are caused is the flip-side of understanding how to cure them. We then go on to explain what 'Bodymind' is and how it works, placing great stress on its protective function. We tell them that, from now on, each time symptoms worsen, they are to pay careful attention to the situations that are going on around them and notice that Bodymind is using symptoms to teaching them something about how to deal with those same situations.

At this point we may also explain how fear of the symptoms, which is created by Headmind, actually makes the symptoms worse as Bodymind picks up that they are in a state of fear and the Hypothalamus triggers fresh symptoms in order to adapt to the new problem. Sometimes, we leave this explanation until later as the cure gets under way should the journal (see below) reveal that fear of the symptoms is indeed a problem.

One of our most important purposes in giving this explanation is to dispel fear of the symptoms. Once clients learn to understand, and trust in, Bodymind's purposes in producing symptoms they are well on the way to doing something about them.

Splitting Bodymind from Headmind. We use a particular style of communication in order to help our clients get more in touch with their personal Bodymind. We first explain that Bodymind, unlike Headmind, doesn't use words and thoughts to communicate. Instead it uses feelings, emotions and symptoms that are experienced in the body and that it may take a little getting used to understanding that symptoms are used by Bodymind as a way of 'talking' to them.

We find analogies and examples are helpful at this point. Some of the ones we use have already been given in Chapter 2, including the 'messenger at the door' analogy. Another is the 'radar' analogy, also given earlier, in which we ask clients to view Bodymind as a super-fast detection system, picking up threats way before we become consciously aware of them, and then using the Hypothalamus to flash a warning signal to let us know in plenty of time that we need to get ready for action. We also give numerous examples of feelings and symptoms from everyday life that tell us that something is wrong. Again, some of these were given in Chapter 2. Another one we use, because it is simple to grasp, is that of someone sitting on a drawing pin. When sitting on a chair with a drawing pin on it, the pin is picked up by the nerve-ends and the signals from the nerves are translated by the brain into a flash of pain that tells the person to get up off the chair quickly. If the symptom is ignored the symptom gets worse until the sufferers eventually gets up. In the same way, Bodymind uses the symptoms of 'Hypothalamitis' to indicate that one particular 'chair' (i.e. an unhealthy situation) will need to be dealt with quickly.

Sensate focusing. Another way we help clients connect to Bodymind communication is to continually direct their attention, using hands and the direction of the voice, to what was going on in the body, in different situations, when symptoms came up. The idea is to sensitise our clients to changes in the body. Understandably, many are afraid of the symptoms or consider them a nuisance and, for that reason, cease to notice when they come and go. In the safe setting of the Reverse Therapy session, we have them recall moments when symptoms came and try to get a feeling of what Bodymind was telling them about the situations they were in at the time. For clients who are unused to sensing bodily changes we may offer them simple exercises in which they hold awareness of different sensations in the body, gradually building up to a deeper awareness of changes in different symptoms.

Setting up the Journal. Reverse Therapy uses journals to record symptoms and the situations connected to them. Once we have helped the client generate the symptom message it is also used to record the actions the client took to respond to the message and what effect this had on reducing symptoms. Journals are *not* used to record thoughts and exercise plans and have nothing in common with the journals used in Cognitive-Behavioural therapy.

Working with symptoms

As I hope this book makes clear, working with symptoms is at the heart of Reverse Therapy. Each and every session concentrates on making clear the underlying symptom-message and encouraging clients to act on it. We also repeat some of the information given in the first session, continually reminding clients about how Bodymind uses the Hypothalamus to produce symptoms, and why it does this. We stress that the symptoms should not be feared but regarded as helpful communications that, if used properly, show the way back to health.

If time permits, and our enquiries yield up sufficient information on the first session, we sometimes go for the symptom message there and then. If not then, once we have gone over the reminders in the second session, we start by looking at what the journal reveals about the link between symptoms and situations. We focus on times when symptoms worsened as well as the occasions when they diminished. The former tells us the problems Bodymind wishes to have changed, while the latter tell us about things clients do that Bodymind approves. For example, a journal might show that symptoms worsened when a client received a visit from her manipulative daughter, who demanded to be allowed to come and live at home again. This indicates that Bodymind is asking for the client to be more forthright about her need for privacy. Another entry might reveal that symptoms lifted when she spent time pottering about in her garden, suggesting that Bodymind is calling for her to use her privacy to spend more time on doing things she loves.

At this stage it is crucial that the Reverse Therapist does not allow her own Headmind to interfere with the process of interpreting the message. In Chapter 4 we looked at some of the most important qualities of the Reverse Therapist and, for me, top of the list should go to the ability to empathise with another person's Bodymind. In doing this, we Reverse Therapists silently ask ourselves the question:

'If I were this person's Bodymind, in this situation, what would I want her to do more of? Less of?'

This question cannot be answered by the Head for the simple reason that Headmind does not have the answers. If it did then clients would not need Reverse Therapy to get well. The fact is that Headmind usually contributes to the problem by blocking, interrupting, de-pressing and explaining away what Bodymind is trying to point to. It does this because it works through fear and conditioning – always demanding that the client do the 'right' thing (right that is, by other people's standards) instead of the 'healthy' thing. If we Reverse Therapists use our Heads to try and work out the symptom message then, we too, will fall into the trap of coming up with answers that fall far short of emotional realities. Remember, also, that Bodymind is sometimes in revolt against Headmind – effectively advising us to ignore it and do something different.

Instead what we do is try and 'tune in' to Bodymind in particular situations, keeping in mind its protective function and its insistence on emotional truth. Personally, I always see Bodymind as a very wise, gifted and innocent child. Like the boy in the fairy-tale it is always ready to announce the obvious fact that the Emperor is wearing no clothes, despite what the crowd thinks.

By degrees, using information from the case history and from the journal, we come closer and closer to helping the client put the symptom-message into words. Using information from the case-history and the Journal, employing empathy and intuition, listening carefully to the client's own choice of words when describing what it was like to endure pressurised situations, the Reverse Therapist generates a symptom message using a card.

Before presenting the client with the message we ask them to focus on the symptoms and try to get a feeling of Bodymind 'talking' them through the symptoms. We then ask them to use the card to put that message into words and read it out aloud.

If the Reverse Therapist has succeeded in getting close to the real message then deep, startling, emotions can be generated as Bodymind responds with a resounding 'Yes!' Typical reactions include:

- A sense of relief.
- Tears.
- Shock (this is Headmind reacting to what it has long denied).
- Sadness.
- Excitement.

It can also sometimes happen that symptoms subside rapidly on reading and digesting the message. This is more likely to occur if the client has one or other of the above emotional reactions, followed by a decision to trust in and abide by Bodymind communication.

Sometimes the message will require some fine-tuning, now or in subsequent sessions, as more information about different pressures and Bodymind needs emerges. Once the message is ready for use we instruct our clients to take three simple steps each time they notice symptoms come up:

1. Focus on the symptoms
2. Read the message
3. Take action immediately in a way that satisfies the message

The journal is then employed in order to note the actions taken, and the effect these had on symptom reduction. Each and every time subsequent sessions open, the journal is consulted in order to monitor progress, fine-tune Bodymind messages and explore other actions (if any were needed) that could have been taken for the situations in question.

Ann's case 2

We first met Ann in Chapter 2, where I described the history of her symptoms and the pressures that forced her Bodymind to produce them. To remind you: her symptoms first appeared when her mother died and she lost an important source of emotional support, with bullying from her sister, cruel treatment from her in-laws, and a lack of support from her husband.

Ann was vaguely aware that these factors 'had something to do with my getting ill' but had yet to make an emotional connection to her Bodymind message.

We worked together on making sense of this until we felt ready to put the message into words.

She then focused on her symptoms of pain and read out the following message:

> *'My symptoms are here to tell me to stop hiding my emotions and start speaking up about them now!'*

Immediately on reading this she became very tearful and began talking about how much she loved and missed her mother. When this conversation had ended, we focused on preparing her for situations that required her to express her emotions.

On the third session, Ann reported that her symptoms had been going up, and then down, 'like a yo-yo'. Her journal showed, predictably, that symptoms had gone up when she took a phone call from her sister, when her in-laws had dropped in one Sunday afternoon, and when her husband one night informed her, without discussion, that he had 'decided' that they would be going on holiday to Cornwall that year.

Her symptoms went rapidly down when she told her husband that if he wanted to go to Cornwall that was his choice but she would not be going and, if he wanted to go on holiday with her, they would need to discuss another destination.

They also went down when she excused herself from her in-laws' company one Sunday and took the dog for a walk.

Her relations with her elder sister took a while to resolve as she had always lived in awe of her but she gradually learned to be more assertive with her and also wrote her a letter expressing her disappointment with her behaviour after mother's death.

She also realised her need for more emotional support. Prior to Reverse Therapy she had been afraid of going out for fear of 'making the symptoms worse' but, with returning confidence, and emotional self-assertion, she spent more and more time going out with her dearest friends (by the end of treatment she was about to embark on a fortnight's holiday with two of them to Minorca).

After eight sessions she was completely well.

Resolving Fear and Depression

These are frequent problems in the treatment of M.E./Chronic Fatigue Syndrome and Fibromyalgia. Fear of the symptoms, as well as fear that one may never get well, actually creates more symptoms as Bodymind picks up that the client is in a state of crisis over their symptoms. It then triggers the Hypothalamus to create more warning signals to the effect that that pressure, too, must be dealt with.

'De-pression', as we call it, has a different root. It is a Headmind reaction that 'de-presses' or disconnects from uncomfortable feelings like fear because they seem overwhelming or just too difficult to deal with. This reaction often accompanies the hopelessness that sets in after years of illness in which little hope of a cure has been offered, and life seems to have become a dull round of pain, exhaustion and disablement.

Sometimes, too, there are other uncomfortable emotions floating around that Headmind tries to de-press. These may include anger (frustration), grief and despair. Some of these may have to do with the experience of illness, while others may have their roots in the original problem in response to which Bodymind was forced to create symptoms. A build up of these emotions, due to their denial or distortion by Headmind, may lead to a 'pressure cooker' effect in which Bodymind struggles to 'keep the lid' on a variety of emotions that, left unexpressed, threaten to explode.

If these emotions are in fact linked to the original pressures then we create a Bodymind symptom-message that encourages clients to be more honest with their emotions and find constructive ways of channelling and expressing them.

If fear and 'de-pression' were caused by the experience of illness, then we adopt a different strategy that we call 'normalisation'. This is a process through which we help clients see that distressing emotions arising from their illness are not strange or peculiar to themselves but normal to anyone who has had to go through the experience they have. We point to the fact that many of our clients tell us about similar feelings that they have, feelings that vanish once they get well. We also point out that Bodymind naturally uses emotions of this kind in order to indicate that a different approach to illness is required as well as to unhelpful people who do not understand the experience of illness. Lastly, we compliment them on having got this far without giving up, and being brave enough to come in for Reverse Therapy. Our strategy is to help build acceptance of their very natural emotions prior to acknowledging and acting on them.

In practice the Reverse Therapy remedy is the same for both Fear and Depression. Since both have their root in a loss of confidence in recovery, the secret is to restore that confidence. Often this arrives when use of the symptom-message acts to reduce symptoms. The sheer joy often reported by clients when this happens is enough to help them on the drive to recovery.

For example, one client, whom I shall call 'Gemma', was working with her symptom-message one day and was asked to do some extra work at the voluntary charity where she worked. Since she had already done more than her fair share of the chores while her co-workers were nowhere to be seen, and her Bodymind message was for her to focus on creating more time for herself, she politely declined and went instead for a walk. Along the way, she noticed that her major symptoms had disappeared! She enjoyed the walk, which took her through one of her favourite parts of the countryside, and, without realising it, walked nearly two miles! Apart from the fact she became a little tired (*not* fatigued) due to the fact she had rarely walked more than a mile in the previous eight years, she felt fine. Before long she was ever more boldly learning to say 'no' to other unreasonable demands on her time while continuing to enjoy her walking, swimming and riding. Within five sessions she was symptom-free.

Other clients may need to take a steadier approach to regain confidence. This is particularly true if they have lived in an atmosphere of fear and doubt for a long time, or if they have lost some of their independence. It may have been a long time since they walked, drove a car, exercised, did the shopping, went to work, or enjoyed an evening out. They may have grown reliant on friends and family members to help them with everyday tasks.

In such cases, we encourage clients to regain their independence by stepping up activities each day, gradually extending the limits for what they do. Since fear of illness carries a secondary chemical memory we often write out a separate symptom-message which reminds them that Bodymind is calling for them to put an end to Fear by regaining their mastery over situations.

Since De-pression typically results from Headmind trying to get rid of Fear by denying it, then once Fear starts to reduce there is no need to de-press feelings. We explain how this 'de-pressing' mechanism works so that clients clearly understand the link between their emotions, their fears and the need to restore confidence. We also work with clients to build in a return to pleasurable activities in their recovery plan. So long as Bodymind is satisfied that they are acting on their message then symptoms can continue to abate. And this, in turn, leaves them free to return to the activities they used to enjoy before their illness.

Increasing the amount of time spent on rewarding pursuits is important in forming new chemical memories. If the old chemical memories were associated with threats, then resolving the threat releases the chemical memory. Since symptoms cannot appear in the absence of a chemical memory, then this also dissolves symptoms, along with the fear and depression that went with struggling to cope with them. If, at the same time, new activities are coming along that bring reward and pleasure, then new chemical memories soon begin to form and quickly replace the old one. A virtuous circle is then set in motion in which new achievement improves confidence, reducing symptoms, bringing new feelings of joy, which still further reduce symptoms...until normal life returns.

What you can do to prepare for your first session

This book is mainly written for people with Chronic Fatigue Syndrome/M.E. and Fibromyalgia who are thinking of coming for Reverse Therapy. If you decide as a result of reading this book that you wish to make an appointment with a Reverse Therapist (please see contact details at the back of this book), then there are a number of things you can do to get ready for your first session.

1. The first is to check that you have a diagnosis of exclusion for your condition. Your GP can advise you on this if you are not sure.

2. Read this book carefully, particularly the key points at the end of each Chapter, and Chapters 5 and 6.

3. Next, consider the history of your symptoms and address the following questions:

    a.   When were the very first appearances of the symptoms, however faint?

    b.   What important pressures were you dealing with at that time?

    c.   What might your Bodymind have been trying to warn you about at that time?

    d.   If symptoms got suddenly worse later on in time, what pressures did you have to deal with then? Again, what was Bodymind trying to warn you about?

    e.   If you have ever had periods when symptoms disappeared or reduced significantly, what circumstances had changed that meant pressures were being resolved? What were you doing at the time that meant Bodymind had less need to warn and protect you from harm?

    4.   Do you notice 'good' days when symptoms improve? What is going on during those days that means Bodymind has less need to communicate to you?

5. Do you notice 'bad' days when symptoms worsen? Again, what situations is Bodymind trying to warn you about on those days?

6. Try to get a 'feel' for your symptoms when they come up and for the Bodymind that works within you. What is this protective presence trying to talk to you about through the symptoms? What would it like you to do?

7. Using this book, reconsider your ideas about CFS/M.E. and Fibromyalgia. Learn to see that your symptoms, however distressing they may appear, have a valuable part to play in your life. They are produced by *your* Bodymind in order to teach you something important. Acknowledging this will make it easier for your Reverse Therapist to work with you on understanding your symptom-message.

8. What does wellness mean to you? If it means simply going back to the pressures that existed before you developed symptoms, you may need to reconsider. Your recovery will ultimately depend on your adoption of a lifestyle that supports wellness. This may mean balancing work with leisure; creating more time to do your own thing; being more emotionally honest with other people; saying 'no' to pressures; and, above all, following activities that bring you inner peace, love, growth and personal fulfilment. Finally, it means being true to yourself and your deepest needs and emotions.

9. If, having read this book, you are still not convinced you can recover, then look harder at the negative effect Headmind may be having on you. It may be that Headmind is filled with hopelessness and despair as a result of the experiences you have gone through. It may also be that you have undergone many 'false dawns' with other treatments that haven't worked and Headmind has concluded that nothing can work. Believe me, I have heard this very often – and most frequently from clients who have gone on to get better! Remember, also, that Headmind tends to believe what everybody else believes. While other people with your

condition may have given up in despair it is vital that you don't – holding close to the lessons in this book, learn to see the deeper, Bodymind, lessons in your symptoms.

Don Colbert and Candace Pert on the emotions of 'bliss'

In their books on Bodymind (see References at the back of this book) both Don Colbert and Candace Pert refer to numerous studies that have demonstrated the profound effects that joy, laughter and pleasure have on neurochemistry.

Different studies have shown that entering into activities that promote bliss – whether this means taking a walk or following a long but rewarding vocation – have the following specific effects:

- Release of Endorphins (the body's mood-boosters)
- Improved Immune system function
- Reduced sensitivity to pain
- Reduction of excess Cortisol
- Lowered blood pressure
- Greater activation of Parasympathetic Nervous System (leading to improved calm, rest and sleep)
- Releases of peptides that form new chemical memories based on satisfaction

This shows that it is just as important to help a client connect to the emotions of joy as it is to help them reduce their Bodymind's need to produce symptoms.

By encouraging involvement in activities that foster these emotions we are aiding Bodymind in its drive to restore balance, deal with pressures, protect and nurture the individual, and promote personal fulfilment.

Key points to remember:

- ➤ Reverse Therapy starts by looking at the environmental pressures that were going on just before symptoms first appeared and, also the pressures continuing in the present

- ➤ Understanding why symptoms are there is the client's first step to recovery

- ➤ Reverse Therapists help clients develop Bodymind awareness so that symptoms can be noticed and understood without fear

- ➤ It is important to prevent Headmind from blocking, interrupting and explaining away Bodymind messages

- ➤ At the core of Reverse Therapy is the art of spelling out symptom-messages so that clients can more easily understand what Bodymind is telling them to do

- ➤ Fear and Depression are resolved by losing fear of 'illness' and restoring confidence gradually through action

- ➤ Side by side with the process of abolishing symptoms by taking action on symptom-messages, clients return to normal life in step-wise fashion

Appendix One

Testimonials

* * *

I had suffered from M.E. for longer than I cared to remember. I had tried every pill, potion, diet, on the planet and spent an absolute fortune. I eventually found a GP who is very sympathetic, though it was not sympathy I required. I read about Reverse Therapy on the web & couldn't stop thinking about 'this miracle cure with no pills or special diet'. I decided to go for it and made an appointment, I had nothing to lose and my life to regain. There was only one drawback 'me country bumpkin', appointment in BIG city – HELP! As the appointment came nearer I was behaving irrationally, not sleeping, eating, ratty (more than usual some would say)! Should I drive in or take the dreaded train aaaggh! I don't do trains, however my urge to get well spurred me on and one glorious May day this year I found myself in the big city. It was no easy task but actually getting myself there alone was a huge step and yes if you'd seen me I was behaving like an escaped mental patient wondering if I'd got on the right train and even worse, was I in the right city?

My first meeting with Dr. Eaton was um interesting, he explained to me how RT worked & what caused Hypothalamitis (or in my case Hippopotamitis because of all the weight I had gained). It all seemed to sink in and I left his office with almost a spring in my step (liar) I was on a strange kind of high but so pleased with myself that I had taken my first step to being normal again. I even managed to get on the right train and soon found myself home. The family gathered round eagerly waiting for news 'well what did he say then?', they asked eagerly. I couldn't remember a thing, total blank, brain in hibernation. 'As mad as a box of frogs' my youngest muttered under her breath...

...However, I started my journal like a dutiful student and soon ran into trouble. An email to John and I was back on track. To start with I found writing my journal hard but soon realised that I was not being honest with myself and had to dig really deep and forget my inhibitions. My next and following appointments were a doddle, I was amazed at my progress and how something so matter of fact could put my life back on track. It's now 6 months since my first appointment and all I have to say is 'I feel great'. I have lost 2½ stones, have regained my self confidence and take a pride in my appearance (I had become a bag lady)! People are amazed at the transformation, which gives me a real buzz. My energy levels are 100% better and I am able to do pretty much what I want. Yes I have the odd bad day – don't we all?

I read my journal regularly just to remind myself what my life was like then and how it is now especially if I'm having a bad day and feeling sorry for myself. I would say to anyone reading this that you have already taken the first step and if you really want to get better contact Reverse Therapy now. I could have easily copped out on the first appointment because of my fear of travelling, panic, anxiety etc. but I knew I had to do it for me. I can never repay Dr Eaton for giving me my life back but if just one person who reads this takes the next step I'll feel like I have done something for all you Hypothalamitis sufferers out there.

SP 2004

* * *

When I first saw Dr Eaton I had had M.E. for 6 years. I could not work at my job and found it very difficult just to get out of bed. In fact I could not do the simplest things like walk down to the shops to buy a newspaper. Everyday life was a nightmare of constant exhaustion, inability to think or concentrate, constant headaches and muscle pain.

I knew that the symptoms could go because there had been two times in my life – both happened while I was away on holiday – when the symptoms left me, only to come back again when I returned to England. That was why I was interested in Reverse therapy because it seemed to have found the secret of making the symptoms go for good.

I was not disappointed. In my case it took three or four sessions before the symptoms started to lift. But Dr Eaton explained to me that my symptoms were with me because my body was trying to warn me and protect me and that it hadn't needed to do that while I was on holiday. What was important was for me to understand what it was about my life here in England that needed to be changed in order for me to get back to health. This I was able to do with Dr Eaton's help.

I am now back at work full time and have no symptoms at all. For me, it is like being on holiday all the time!

NF 2004

* * *

I was 32 going on 62 and had given up hope of any sort of recovery or return to my normal life. I had decided that I was better off without all alternative therapy cures that promised so much, but did nothing for me or even made me worse. But when I read about RT a light bulb clicked on in my head, telling me this could be the answer. I had to try it. That was only a year ago but it feels like a lifetime away.

Incredibly, I'm now back at work, enjoying a social life and making positive plans for the future. I consider myself to be fully recovered. My symptoms started to lift at my very first appointment, immediately upon reading my first message. The therapy was sometimes hard work and emotionally draining, but I was always rewarded with a lifting of symptoms. Thanks to the commitment and understanding of my therapist, Reverse Therapy has been an unforgettable and life changing experience, and one that I recommend to all ME sufferers.

SH 2004

* * *

I was in the depths of despair over my condition before I came for R.T. From not being able to do the slightest task I am now back to having a normal life. Thank you to R.T. for giving me my health back.

R M 2003

* * *

I am writing to let you know that I haven't had any symptoms since I saw you. Not only have the tiredness etc not recurred, but my sleep is improving (not fast enough!) and listening to the symptoms helped, and also my allergic reactions to foods have all but disappeared. Long may the force be with you.

R Mc 2003

* * *

I was an M.E. sufferer for many years; no energy, memory loss, body clock out of order and above all very severe muscle spasms which required three 5mg Diazepam tablets daily.

I had four consultations in which it was explained to me that M.E. was the result of a dysfunctional Hypothalamus gland also what I was required to do to encourage this gland to function properly again.

I am a new man and have not had a spasm in the last five months. Energy, memory and concentration have all greatly improved.

I can't thank Reverse Therapy enough. I will be forever grateful to them for giving me a new lease of life.

JB 2004

* * *

I have had Post Viral Fatigue for 12 years with restricted mobility, have never been bed-bound but sometimes, at the beginning, house-bound. I have tried numerous complementary therapies, all of which helped with the symptoms but did not, and did not claim to, cure the illness.

In December last year I was asked by another member of the group if I had heard of Reverse Therapy. After some investigations and being in email contact with someone who found all her symptoms had disappeared using the technique, I decided to give it a try.

After the first session I was able to banish my brain fog for at least an hour and was so thrilled that I danced round the kitchen, a physical impossibility a week before.

Over the next few weeks I have seen all my symptoms disappear, with slight re-occurrences which I am again able to get rid of with my message and my reaction to it.

I used to pace my activities and have at least three rests a day, I rarely need one rest now. Only three times in the last six months have I had that dreadful exhaustion which used to be a regular occurrence after any excursion and never during this time have I felt that I was going to have a relapse.

Reverse Therapy is an incredible idea, but it has worked for me and for many others. I like to say that it has given me permission to do things again, to live a normal life. It really is worth looking into.

JM 2004

* * *

I travelled from the South-West of France to see Dr John Eaton and knew immediately that Reverse Therapy was the missing link in my battle with M.E..

In just one hour John had removed the fear from my life and began to teach me how to listen to my body. I now knew I could concentrate on getting well instead of worrying about being ill.

It's been an amazing experience that has completely transformed my life, not just physically but emotionally as well.

Reverse Therapy works. You should try it; you have nothing to lose and so much to gain.

CB 2004

Appendix Two

Contacting a Reverse therapist

Dr John Eaton has set up Reverse Therapy UK in order to provide ethical, supervised treatment with professionally trained practitioners who are committed to the relief of illness, wherever they may find it. He strongly advises readers to utilise the services of practitioners registered with Reverse Therapy UK who use this trade-marked logo and who are authorised to issue a Reverse Therapy UK Registration Number:

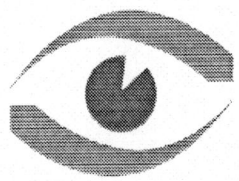

REVERSE THERAPY

Although this book provides detailed information about the process of Reverse Therapy it is strongly recommended that you work with a trained practitioner in order to get well. This is because, with the best will in the world, it can be difficult to reverse the effects of Headmind attitudes to symptoms and reach an emotionally honest view of Bodymind symptom-messages, without the help of a Reverse Therapist.

Having said that, Dr Eaton would be extremely interested to learn from anyone who has succeeded in becoming symptom-free simply with the aid of this book and you can contact him through any of the addresses given below.

Reverse Therapy UK can be contacted in a variety of ways:

➢ Through our website: www.reverse-therapy.com
➢ Through email: info@reverse-therapy.com
➢ Through our telephone line: 01635 44444 (Answer phone service only)

> Through our postal address:
Waterloo House, 158 London Rd, Newbury, Berkshire, UK, RG14 AX

Appendix Three

Research supporting 'Hypothalamitis'

Research carried out over the past fifteen years or so has abundantly shown up the central role of the Hypothalamus/HPA axis in creating the symptoms. Here are some of the more important findings:

- Lowered production of Cortisol due to impaired function of the HPA axis in CFS/M.E. and FMS sufferers compared with a control group of non-sufferers.

- CFS patients demonstrated over-stimulation of the Sympathetic Nervous System dysfunction, caused by HPA axis dysfunction.

- Individuals with Chronic Fatigue Syndrome showed increased Prolactin release, a hormone released by the Pituitary gland, under the control of the Hypothalamus. The main function of Prolactin is to boost milk production in women but it also has an important secondary role in regulating the Immune system.

- Groups of Chronic Fatigue Syndrome patients were shown to have marked impairment of Adrenal function, including, in some advanced cases, shrunken Adrenal glands.

- Changes in hormonal activities regulated by the Hypothalamus leading to increased sensitivity to pain have been identified as a leading trigger for the symptoms experienced by Fibromyalgia sufferers.

- Disorders in both the Sympathetic Nervous System and in the HPA axis (leading to reduced production of Cortisol) were found in women patients with Fibromyalgia.

- CFS patients undergoing stress tests had lower AcTH response levels (AcTH is produced by the Pituitary gland on instructions from the Hypothalamus and acts to stimulate the Adrenal glands) leading to abnormalities in Cortisol production.

Concerning this last finding, it is important to note that some researchers believe that the Hypothalamus is *underactive* in CFS/M.E. In Reverse therapy we consider that the Hypothalamus is generally (but not always specifically) overactive, thus producing the condition we term 'Hypothalamitis'.

This hypothesis is supported by the fact that many symptoms – muscle weakness, fatigue, gut problems, pain and circulatory problems, point to over-work of major body functions. The fact that symptoms can be reversed spontaneously also points to over-activity in the Central Nervous System, which can quickly be corrected, rather than to a failure in glandular function.

There are two main reasons why the Hypothalamus *appears* to be underactive:

1. Exhaustion of the Adrenal glands, resulting in a failure to respond to signals from the Hypothalamus-Pituitary (e.g. AcTH releases).

2. Breakdown in the control exercised, through feedback, by the Hypothalamus over the Immune system and, also, the Adrenal glands.

In both cases this points to an under-responsiveness on the part of the Adrenal glands, *not* under-activity in the Hypothalamus.

Appendix Four

References and further reading

Chapter 1

Milton Erickson. *The Collected Papers of Milton Erickson*. 1980.
Eugene Gendlin. *Focusing*. 1982.
Stephen Gilligan. *Therapeutic Trances*. 1987
Ernest Rossi. *The Psychobiology of Mind-Body Healing*. 1986.
Ernest Rossi. *The Symptom Path to Enlightenment*. 1996.

Chapter 2

William Blake. *Songs of Innocence and Experience, The Marriage of Heaven and Hell, and The Everlasting Gospel*.
(Blake is an excellent guide to Bodymind wisdom as well as the dangers of over-relying on Headmind!)
Henry Dreher. *Mind-Body Unity*. 2003.
Ken Dychtwald. *Bodymind*. 1977.
John Eaton and Roy Johnson. *Communicate with Emotional Intelligence*. 2001.
Daniel Goleman. *Emotional Intelligence*. 1996.
Fritz Perls. *Gestalt Therapy Verbatim*. 1969.

Chapter 3

Don Colbert. *Deadly Emotions*. 2003.
Ryke-Geerd Hamer. His main work '*Vermächtnis einer Neuen Medizin*' has not yet been translated into English . Information on Hamer's work in English is on the following website: http://www.neue-medizin/hamereng.htm
Joseph LeDoux. *The Emotional Brain*. 1999.
Paul Martin. *The Sickening Mind*. 1997.
Candace Pert. *Molecules of Emotion*. 1997.
Hans Selye. *The Stress of Life*. 1978.
Esther Sternberg & Philip Gold. *The Mind-Body Interaction in Disease*. (Scientific American – Special Issue). 1997.

Chapter 5

Henri. F. Ellenberger. *The Discovery of The Unconscious*. 1994.
David W. Jameson. *Mind-Body Health and Stress Tolerance*. 2003
Lauren B. Krupp. *Fatigue*. 2003.
Dr Charles Shepherd. *Living with M.E.* 1999.
D. J. Wallace and J. B. Wallace. *Fibromyalgia*. 2003
James L. Wilson. *Adrenal Fatigue*. 2001.

Chapter 6

William Hudson O'Hanlon and Michele Weiner-Davies. *In Search of Solutions*. 1989.